KT-133-234

A Waldorf Guide to
Children's Health

Illnesses, Symptoms, Treatments and Therapies

Dr Michaela Glöckler
Dr Wolfgang Goebel
Dr Karin Michael

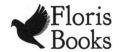

Floris
Books

Translated by Catherine Creeger

The section 'Diabetes' was written
by Dr Dörte Hilgard, specialist in children's diabetics at
Herdecke Hospital in Germany. The chapter 'External
Treatments for Home Nursing' was written by Petra Lange

Originally published in German under the title
Kindersprechstunde by Verlag Urachhaus in 1984
First published in English in 1990 by Floris Books, Edinburgh
as *A Guide to Child Health*
Fifth edition published in 2018, translated and adapted
from the twenty-first German edition of 2017

© 1984, 2017 Verlag Freies Geistesleben & Urachhaus GmbH
English version © 2018 Floris Books, Edinburgh

All rights reserved. No part of this publication may be
reproduced in any form without the written permission of
Floris Books, Edinburgh
www.florisbooks.co.uk

British Library CIP data available
ISBN 978-178250-529-7
Printed in Malta by Gutenberg

Emergency Contents

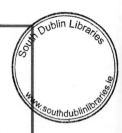

A list of emergencies and common childhood concerns is given below as a quick reference, to help you easily find the appropriate page for guidance. **If in doubt, always call the emergency services or take your child to your nearest hospital.**

South Dublin Libraries
www.southdublinlibraries.ie

Note

The information in this book is based on years of clinical practice and study, and every effort has been made to present it in a clear and reliable manner.

Where the information is medical in nature, please be aware that medicines available on prescription will vary from country to country. Also, names of some medicines are different in some countries.

Anthroposophic medicine is a complementary medicine that seeks to extend, not replace, mainstream medicine. The authors and publisher warn that readers should not rely on the content of this book as a substitute for conventional medical treatment. The applications and case studies described here cannot replace the advice of a medical specialist. When diagnosing and managing specific health conditions, always seek the advice of your doctor/physician.

Contents

Pleasure is a gift of destiny
that reveals its value in the present,
while suffering is a source of insight
whose significance will become evident in the future.

Rudolf Steiner

Preface

A *Waldorf Guide to Children's Health* aims to encourage parents, especially young parents, to develop confidence in dealing with their children both in illness and health. It may also be useful for childcare practitioners, healthcare workers, therapists and doctors who want to learn more about a holistic approach to paediatrics and an integrative approach to anthroposophic medicine in paediatrics. This book is the result of decades of experience: the authors are former or current doctors of the children's department of Herdecke Clinic in Germany, the largest anthroposophic hospital in the world. Since this book's first appearance in German in 1984 it has been translated into 23 languages, and we are happy to see that our experience is benefiting a growing number of children. This English-language edition has been revised to cover a variety of therapeutic applications and suggestions, and to focus the book on practical medical advice.

Integrative medicine looks at human development in terms of body, soul and spirit, as well as modern psychology and influences from the environment, to draw appropriate conclusions for diagnosis and treatment of various diseases. This is made possible both by Rudolf Steiner's anthroposophy and by salutogenesis, a medical approach focusing on preventative factors that support human health and well-being rather than focusing primarily on the causes of disease.

The early chapters of this book are devoted to first aid and common childhood illnesses, helping parents to recognise specific symptoms and problems, and take appropriate therapeutic measures. Our intention is to help parents who are observing and supporting sick children to determine when a visit to the doctor is either absolutely necessary or advisable as a precautionary measure. For the most part we have limited our therapeutic recommendations to very general measures to avoid impinging on a doctor's freedom to decide what is best in each individual case. The later chapters are more contemplative, offering advice on subjects such as caring for babies, the importance of rhythm for physical and mental health, preventing illness and vaccination.

Although there is no chapter on screen time in this edition, we would like to make a special plea to support the healthy development of the next generation by avoiding the tendency of 'earlier and faster' which the rapid increase in digital technology is promoting, even among the youngest in our society. Development takes time; the brain is a delicate organ that needs to relate to the real world and its objects in order to develop in a healthy way.

We would like to thank Wolfgang Goebel, who originally had the idea for this book and, until the beginning of this century, used his knowledge and paediatric experience to bring every new edition up to date. Our thanks also go to parents and colleagues who have repeatedly provided us with suggestions and feedback for improving our presentation. Last but not least, we thank our publisher Floris Books for making the 21st edition of this book available in the English-speaking world.

Michaela Glöckler, 2018

1. First Aid and Accidents

Children are naturally motivated by the joy of discovery, but parents should be aware that this curiosity can also lead to accidents, especially with toddlers. It is common for children to get a fright when an accident occurs, but they recover most quickly from the shock in the presence of an adult who can take stock of the situation rationally, keep calm and take rapid action. These qualities are vital in order to be truly helpful. Getting angry or offering exaggerated expressions of sympathy make the situation more difficult for children, even if their own actions caused the accident.

▶ The advice we offer here is no substitute for a course in first aid, and we urge all readers to take such a course.

1.1 Resuscitation

Mouth-to-mouth resuscitation

Lay the child on their back and tip the head back by pressing on the forehead and lifting the chin (if the child is under 1 year old, the head should be straight). Cover the open mouth and nose of an infant with your own lips; with older children, pinch the nose shut and breathe into the mouth only. Take a deep breath, then blow 5 times, carefully, so that the child's ribcage rises and falls each time. If the mouth is injured, resuscitation can also be done mouth-to-nose.

Heart massage (CPR)

Applying short strokes of firm pressure to the breastbone (approximately 2 strokes per second), using both thumbs for infants (adapt the pressure to the elasticity of the infant ribcage) or the ball of your hand for older children.

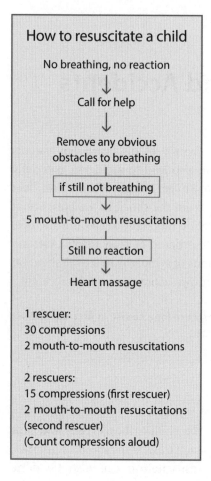

How to resuscitate a child

No breathing, no reaction

↓

Call for help

↓

Remove any obvious
obstacles to breathing

|

if still not breathing

↓

5 mouth-to-mouth resuscitations

|

Still no reaction

↓

Heart massage

1 rescuer:
30 compressions
2 mouth-to-mouth resuscitations

2 rescuers:
15 compressions (first rescuer)
2 mouth-to-mouth resuscitations
(second rescuer)
(Count compressions aloud)

If you are alone, call for help after 1 minute of resuscitation. Otherwise ask someone else to call for help. Give your name and address (including the location in building).

How to resuscitate a baby

- If a baby is lying pale and motionless in bed and is not breathing visibly, briefly hold their head down to allow any vomit or phlegm out of the mouth. If necessary, gently tap your baby's back with your fingers.

- Check your baby's mouth for remaining vomit or tough phlegm that may be blocking the airways. Immediately wipe out the mouth and throat with your little finger.

- Move your baby as quickly as possible to a hard surface (table, bench, floor).

- Immediately begin **mouth-to-mouth resuscitation** followed by **heart massage** (see page 13).

Further Advice

- These measures will be effective only if the respiratory arrest has been brief.

- As soon as you feel a heartbeat or pulse, stop the cardiac massage and continue mouth-to-mouth resuscitation until the child is breathing on their own again. **However, do not waste unnecessary time checking for a pulse.**

- Resuscitation attempts are easier if 1 person performs the heart massage and another the mouth-to-mouth resuscitation.

- Of course these techniques are most effective if performed by someone who has received training in a first-aid course. **Nonetheless, an untrained person should also immediately attempt to implement these measures** because they are the only chance of bringing the child back to life. Those present in situations of extreme danger must do whatever they can to help.

- A possible complication of resuscitation attempts is that the stomach can also inflate because of air blown into the oesophagus. If this happens, periodically attempt to press the air out of the child's abdomen with your hand.
- Other complications may result if excessive force is used either in inflating the lungs (pulmonary rupturing) or applying cardiac massage (broken ribs). The possibility of such complications must not deter anyone from attempting resuscitation if there is no prospect of emergency medical personnel reaching the scene immediately. If the child is still breathing but is gasping for breath or breathing irregularly, try clapping on their cheeks, back and the side of the ribcage to see if the situation improves.
- Even if the child recovers rapidly and returns to normal, get professional advice as soon as possible.

1.2 Choking and suffocation

Causes
- Aspiration of vomit into the windpipe, which usually occurs only in very young infants or children who are not fully conscious.
- A piece of a nut or a part of a toy 'goes down the wrong way' and is inhaled rather than swallowed. This happens mainly to toddlers, but anyone can be at risk.

Symptoms
- Sudden coughing
- Gagging
- Difficulty breathing
- Strange noises while breathing
- Child turns blue
- In less acute cases, ongoing coughing or even pneumonia

Action
▶ **If your child cannot breathe, cannot cough or turns dark blue, but is STILL CONSCIOUS**

- Shout for help but do not leave your child.
- Carefully search their mouth for the object, making sure not to push it further down.
- Use back blows.
- Then chest or abdominal thrusts.
- Call emergency services.

Back blows

Place **babies under 1 year** face down on your forearm or thighs with 1 hand supporting their head.

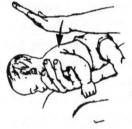

Place **toddlers and older children** face down over your knee, with 1 hand supporting their head. Their head and torso should tilt downwards.

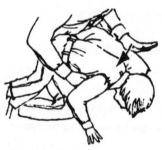

With your free hand, clap their back between the shoulder blades up to 5 times.

If the object has not been expelled and your child is still conscious, give chest or abdominal thrusts.

Chest or abdominal thrusts

Carefully turn **babies under 1 year** on their back and lay them on your thighs, keeping their body at the same downwards tilting angle. Place 2 fingers in the middle of the sternum and give sharp chest thrusts up to 5 times.

For **children over 1 year**, stand or kneel behind them, wrap your arms around them, place a fist between their navel and ribs and pull forcefully inwards and upwards, up to 5 times.

If the object is still stuck

- Repeat the sequence of back blows and chest or abdominal compressions.
- Call or send out for help but do not leave your child.

▶ If your child is not breathing and UNCONSCIOUS

- Lay them on a flat surface.
- Shout for help but do not leave your child.
- Call emergency services.
- If you can see the obstacle to breathing, remove it.
- Start resuscitation, with 5 mouth-to-mouth breaths and heart massage (see page 13).

▶ If your child can still breathe

- Call emergency services.
- Do not drive your child to the hospital yourself.
- Do not pat your child on the back and do not place them head-down.
- Do not give your child anything to eat or drink.

- Accompany your child in the ambulance.

Prevention

- Grind nuts for toddlers; do not allow them to eat larger pieces. Children under the age of 5 should not be given whole nuts, or be allowed to play with marbles or toys with small parts that can be removed or bitten off. Avoid too much silliness and joking around at mealtimes. Choking can be dangerous.
- Be aware that small children can accidentally strangle themselves on cords or chains, especially where these are stretched across a pram or bed. Plastic bags are not toys; they can cause suffocation.
- Remember that warning children can simply encourage them to do what's forbidden, so stay alert and make sure that your children's surroundings are safe.

1.3 Drowning

- Lower the child's head to let any water run out.
- **If the child is not breathing**, begin mouth-to-mouth resuscitation (see page 13) immediately and perform heart massage if needed (see page 13). Take a first-aid course to learn the technique, but an untrained person should also attempt these live-saving measures straightaway.
- Provide pure oxygen as soon as possible.

1.4 Traffic accidents

- If the injured child is **still breathing, speaking and moving**, lay them on their side, cover them warmly and stay with them until help arrives. Due to shock they will probably be pale and may vomit.
- If the child is **unconscious but still breathing**, do not move them until trained help arrives. Cover them warmly and stay with them if possible.
- If the child **is not breathing**, give mouth-to-mouth resuscitation immediately. If they have no pulse or heartbeat, administer cardiac massage to the best of your ability.
- If the child is **bleeding heavily**, cover spurting blood or a steady flow with the cleanest cloth available and apply pressure. Do not apply a tourniquet. Slight bleeding will stop by itself.
- If the child is **in severe pain**, do not move them (this is especially important for back pain). Moving the victim can cause further damage.

- If the child has **minor injuries**, the quickest way to find out where they are hurt is to ask them to move each limb by themselves. Help them very carefully.
- **Call emergency services in all these cases.**

1.5 Allergic (anaphylactic) shock

This can be life-threatening, so be aware of the triggers and be prepared to act quickly.

Triggers
- Medicines
- Food
- Insect bites

Warning signs
- Nausea and vomiting
- Raised, itchy skin rash (also called nettle rash or hives)
- Swelling, dryness or tingling of mucous membranes (e.g. the openings of the eyes, ears, mouth and nose)
- Breathing difficulties (similar to asthma symtoms)

Symptoms
- Escalation of warning signs
- Pallor (i.e. unusual paleness of skin compared to your child's usual complexion)
- Breathing difficulties
- Unconsciousness
- Cardiac arrest

Action
- Call emergency services immediately.
- If available (with high-risk children), use an emergency adrenaline auto-injector.
- If necessary, resuscitate (see page 13).

1.6 Fainting

Causes
- Standing for a long time
- Stuffy atmosphere
- Pain
- Reaction to the sight of blood

Symptoms
- Pallor (i.e. unusual paleness of skin compared to your child's usual complexion)
- Heavy breathing
- Breaking out in a sweat
- Collapse
- Unconsciousness

Action
- Lie the unconscious child on the ground and elevate their legs.
- Loosen tight clothing and belts.
- Ensure there is fresh air.
- A whiff of an aromatic substance (e.g. rosemary) may help.

- Sponge their face with cool water.
- Once the child has recovered sufficiently to safely swallow, give Weleda Cardiodoron (5–10 drops in some water).

1.7 Breath-holding attacks

Causes

With some children, sudden screams of pain or anger may be followed by momentary loss of consciousness. There are two types: 'blue breath-holding attacks' and 'reflex anoxic seizures'.

Symptoms

- *Blue breath-holding attacks:* these can occur if your child is very upset and sobbing. Your child may turn blue and stop breathing, but breathing will start again after they gasp or take a breath in.
- *Reflex anoxic seizure:* these can occur if your child has a sudden fright (the trigger may or may not be clear). Your child might not cry; typically they will turn pale-grey and lose consciousness. While unconscious, they will be stiff and gasp when they come around and colour comes back into their face.

Action

- Remain calm. The more upset adults become, the more likely it is that the incident will be repeated, because children instinctively sense the impact of their condition on adults.
- Lie your child on their side and watch them until the attack is over.
- Ensure your child cannot hit their head or limbs on anything surrounding them.
- Do not shake them.
- Do not put anything in their mouth.
- Do not splash them with water.
- Do not attempt mouth-to-mouth resuscitation – the attack should subside on its own, usually in under a minute.
- Consult a doctor if more than a few such incidents occur.

1.8 Toxic and corrosive substances

We all have dangerous substances in and around our houses including acids (toilet cleaner), bases (ammonia, caustic soda and bleaching agents), corrosive substances (polish, spray cleaner and gasoline), and toxic substances (medicines, alcohol, some plants).

Eye injuries from acids or bases

- Rinse the affected eye under lightly running cool water for approximately 10 minutes, making sure the eye is fully opened.
- Then take your child to the nearest hospital Accident and Emergency department.

Skin burns caused by corrosive substances

- Remove clothing quickly.
- Rinse the affected area thoroughly under running water, then treat as for burns (see page 21).

Swallowing acids or bases

- If your child swallows acids, bases or any corrosive substances, such as polish, spray cleaner or gasoline, **do not induce vomiting**, which would expose the oesophagus to the corrosive substance again. Instead, **immediately give your child plenty of water or tea to dilute the poison**.
- **Do not give milk,** as it absorbs the poisonous substances rather than diluting them, allowing them to get into the bloodstream more quickly.
- Head for your nearest hospital Accident and Emergency department.

Swallowing pills, alcohol or non-corrosive poisons

Symptoms

- Drowsiness
- Unusual excitability
- Vomiting
- Diarrhoea
- Stomach pain
- Pain in or around your child's mouth
- Fever
- Headache
- Loss of appetite
- Difficulty swallowing
- Dribbling
- Irregular breathing
- Blue lips and skin
- Skin rash
- Seizures
- Becoming unconscious or unresponsive

Action

- If you suspect poisoning, **call emergency services** or **head for your nearest hospital Accident and Emergency department**.
- If you can't get medical help quickly, **induce vomiting at home as soon possible**.
- *In any case of suspected poisoning,* search your child's surroundings for empty or unsealed packages of medication, bottles of solvents, unfamiliar plant parts etc. Take this and any vomit (induced or spontaneous) with you to the hospital.

How to induce vomiting

- Give your child 2–4 cups of water to drink (add fruit juice, if readily available, to improve the taste).
- Hold a **small child** over your knee; an **older child** should lie on their side.
- With 1 hand, press your child's cheeks in between opened teeth. With the index finger of the other hand, touch the back of the throat (or insert the handle of a spoon into the throat) until vomiting begins.

Prevention

- Keep all domestic fluids, poisons and medicines locked up out of reach of children.
- Keep health centre posters or local authority advice on poisons and stings at hand as well. Your local poison information centres can be found online and in telephone directories.

1.9 Burns and scalds

Action

Major burns and scalds

- If more than 15% of the body's surface has been burned, **immediately call emergency services**, as the consequences of cooling can be worse than the scalding.

A child with burns covering more than 5% of the body's surface must be hospitalised for observation, because generalised symptoms can develop over the next few days. **As a point of reference, the surface of a child's hand is approximately 1% of their body surface.**

- If sensitive body parts are affected (eyes or face), **immediately consult a doctor**.
- **Immediately pour cold water** (cold tap water, not iced) over the affected areas. Hold the area under cold (preferably running) water for not more than 10–15 minutes.
- If the clothing is not stuck to the skin, undress your child. It is particularly important to remove any clothing if your child was scalded by oil.
- If you act quickly, cold water can prevent blistering and serious skin damage.
- Cover any blisters with a clean (sterile or freshly ironed) cloth and consult a doctor.

Minor burns and scalds

- Smaller burns can be treated at home. Keep the wound constantly moist with Weleda Combudoron ointment or Weleda Burns & Bites Cooling Gel (diluting with boiled water if necessary).
- Do not break open blisters.

- After a day or two, allow the burn or scald to air-dry. If necessary, cover it with a dry bandage.

1.10 Head injuries

Minor head injuries
Causes

Young children often fall and knock their heads, for instance, a toddler may roll off a low bed onto a carpeted floor with a bump, or infants may crash their heads together while playing.

Symptoms

- Cries immediately
- Does not vomit
- Cushion-like swellings on their skull; feel their head straightaway, and again half an hour later
- As soon as your child recovers from the shock, they are quite lively again

Action

- Press the ball of your hand against the affected area or apply a cold washcloth for 5 minutes.
- Apply arnica essence or ointment if there is swelling.
- There is no need for a doctor to examine your child if the injury is minor.

More serious head injuries
Causes

If your baby falls off the changing table or out of their highchair, or an older child falls from a climbing frame or swing and hits their head on a hard surface, you should seek medical advice.

Symptoms

- Loss of consciousness (even if only briefly)
- Difficulty staying awake or keeping their eyes open
- Vision problems
- Vomiting
- A cushion-like swelling on their skull (possible skull fracture)
- Clear fluid coming from their ears or nose
- Bleeding from their ears or bruising behind their ears
- Numbness or weakness in their body
- Problems with balance, understanding, speaking or writing
- Seizures or fits
- **If your child shows none of the above symptoms but you are still concerned, seek medical advice.**

Action

- Take your child immediately to your nearest hospital Accident and Emergency department.

1.11 Nosebleeds

Action

- If the nosebleed was caused by a fall, if the bridge of the nose swells or if the nose appears deformed, call your doctor.
- Sit your child down leaning against the back of a chair but with their head bent slightly forwards.
- Press with 2 fingers (or a cool washcloth) against both sides of their nose (where no bone gets in the way) to close both nostrils.
- After 5 minutes, let go, ask your child to blow their nose and wait to see if bleeding recurs. Repeat the process if needed.
- If the bleeding does not stop within 10 minutes, call your doctor.

1.12 Swallowing a foreign object

- If something like a marble, coin or paperclip is swallowed, it usually passes through the system without causing damage. To be sure it has passed through your child's body safely, search your child's stools carefully by breaking them up in water in a potty. But always seek urgent medical attention if your child swallows:

- An object larger than 2 cm (¾ in) in diameter: they often get stuck, usually in the oesophagus or in the throat, leading to a blockage of air passages.
- A sharp object.
- A small battery: they contain corrosives and may cause serious stomach damage.

Symptoms

- Choking, difficulty swallowing
- Increased salivation
- Nausea, vomiting
- Stomachache

Action

- If the object swallowed is round and there is a blockage of air passages, call emergency services immediately and, if necessary, proceed as in acute danger of suffocation (see page 15).

1.13 Cuts and grazes

Serious injuries

Always seek medical help for the following:

- Gaping wounds and puncture wounds
- Wounds that continue to bleed
- Animal and human bites that puncture the skin
- Insect bites in the throat or back of the mouth. For insect bites, give your child a cold drink

to sip or ice to suck on and see a doctor immediately.

Tetanus prevention

When unvaccinated children are cut by dirty objects, are bitten or are stung by a wasp or other insect that is in frequent contact with the ground, they can be at risk of contracting tetanus. It is important to seek medical advice. For more information, see Section 14.3, page 264.

Small, bleeding cuts

- Before cleaning, wash your hands and dry them on a clean towel.
- Allow the wound to bleed for a few minutes.
- Rinse the wound with lukewarm water.
- Apply a sterile adhesive or gauze bandage, or simply leave the wound to air-dry.

Scrapes (abrasions) on the knees

- Before cleaning, wash your hands and dry them on a clean towel.
- Carefully clean the scrape using cooled, boiled water and sterile gauze or an ironed cloth.
- Scrapes should be allowed to air-dry.
- If necessary, apply a thick layer of an antiseptic powder.

- Use a bandage or plaster to prevent further injury and to protect the scrape from rubbing against clothing. Change as necessary.

Oozing wounds

- Treat slightly oozing infected wounds with an antiseptic powder.
- Treat heavily oozing infected wounds twice daily with a thick layer of antiseptic ointment to prevent them from sticking to the bandage. If you are concerned, seek medical advice.

1.14 Other common injuries

Splinters, thorns and ticks

Remove them from the skin as soon as possible. To remove a tick, lift it out of the skin carefully with a needle or with a pair of tick tweezers (available from your pharmacy), using an anticlockwise twisting motion as you pull it out. If part of the tick remains in the skin, consult your doctor (see Section 14.2, page 281).

Crushed finger

When a finger has been crushed in a door or similar, hold it under cold running water for

3–5 minutes. Depending on the severity of the injury, either apply a bandage moistened with arnica essence or consult a doctor immediately.

Tooth knocked out

Take both your child *and* the tooth to a dentist immediately. Keep the tooth moist in a sterile saline solution (cooking salt mixed with water). Try not to touch the broken surface or the root of the tooth.

2. Pain

The younger the child, the more difficult it is to find out where it hurts. For this reason, common pain-causing ailments and injuries will all be discussed in one chapter to show to what extent parents can recognise what is causing the pain.

Children's reactions to pain depend in part on the circumstances that surround them. As adults, we are called upon to support our children by responding with composure and confidence. If we ourselves can face the situation calmly, our children will tolerate pain differently than if we panic. Children pick up on our agitation, anxiety or long-winded expressions of sympathy, which simply intensify their experience of pain.

2.1 Headaches

Meningitis

There are two types of meningitis, viral and bacterial, and the symptoms are similar.

- **Viral meningitis** is usually less dangerous than bacterial meningitis. But there are also severe forms (e.g. measles or herpesis) that may need hospitalisation and possibly antiviral treatment.
- **Bacterial (septic) meningitis**, caused by a bacterial infection, can be much more serious.

If you suspect meningitis, **immediately take your child to your nearest hospital Accident and Emergency department**, where a lumbar puncture (using a fine needle to extract spinal fluid for further testing) can be performed. Prompt antibiotic treatment very often prevents permanent damage from bacterial meningitis, but this condition and its treatment require hospitalisation.

Symptoms
- Persistent and very severe headache
- Blotchy rash that does not fade when a glass is rolled over it
- Frequently a high fever
- Feeling sick and vomiting

- Irritability
- Lack of energy
- Aching muscles and joints
- Stiff neck
- Breathing rapidly
- Cold hands and feet
- Pallor (unusual paleness of skin compared to your child's usual complexion) and mottled skin
- Confusion
- Dislike of bright lights
- Drowsiness
- Fits or seizures

Babies might also:
- Refuse feeds
- Have a stiff body
- Be floppy or unresponsive
- Not want to be picked up
- Have a bulging fontanelle (soft spot towards the front of their head)
- Have an unusual high-pitched cry

Action

You can perform the following tests to see if meningitis is a possibility, but **if you are in any doubt, take your child to your nearest hospital Accident and Emergency department.**

How to check for meningitis

- Ask your child to lift their arms while sitting on the bed with legs outstretched. Do they have to support themselves from behind? If they cannot do this without pain and have to support themselves, seek urgent medical help.
- In a sitting position, can your child kiss their knee by bending their neck and flexing their knee until they can touch it with their mouth? Pain and neck stiffness arising from meningitis would prevent children from raising their knee to their chin. If your child cannot do this, seek urgent medical help.

Being able to perform both of these movements virtually rules out the possibility of meningitis. Be aware, though, that a child may baulk, start to cry and appear unable to perform if parents seem unduly anxious or over-explain their request.

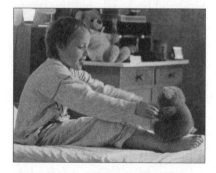

Figure 1. This child definitely does not have meningitis. He can sit with his arms extended, bending forward from the hips with legs outstretched, without feeling pain.

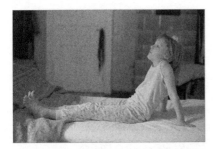

Figure 2. Meningitis is probable in this case. When asked to sit up and keep her knees straight, this girl supports herself from behind and keeps her head bent somewhat backwards. She cannot extend her arms forward without pain.

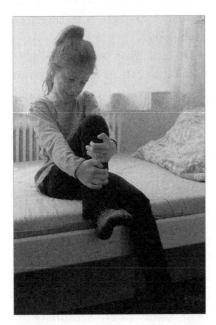

Figure 3. Pain and neck stiffness also prevent her from raising her knee to her chin or kissing it, even when she uses her arms to help. If your child cannot perform this gesture, meningitis or at least meningeal irritation is even more probable, and prompt examination by a doctor is advised.

If your child is too young for such tests or fails either one of them, or if you are in any doubt, take your child to your nearest hospital Accident and Emergency department.

Urgent treatment requires hospitalisation, but your continued presence beside your child is very important.

Myogelosis

Note that myogelosis, or muscular contraction or inflammation of the lymph nodes located deep in the neck, can produce similar symptoms to meningitis. Always seek medical help if you are concerned. (See page 39 for more information on myogelosis.)

Headaches with a rising fever
Cause

Onset of a fever due to a cold, flu or other illness; the headache usually disappears once the fever peaks.

Symptoms
- Exhaustion
- Loss of appetite
- Aching limbs
- General malaise
- Shivering
- Headache
- Stomachache
- Nausea
- Later, fever of 39.5°C (103°F) or over

Action

- If your child still feels cold, they need to be warmed up, beginning with their feet (give them wool socks to wear).
- Ensure a peaceful, low-stimulus environment.
- Give your child some warm herb tea (without caffeine) such as lemon balm, lightly sweetened if desired.
- Children who are developing a fever do not need to eat; if they ask for food, give them something light.
- Many children appreciate a cool hand, a light silk cloth or a damp washcloth on their forehead.
- If your child starts to show symptoms of meningitis as outlined above, or if you are concerned about your child, seek medical help.
- **Always consult your doctor if a headache or vomiting persists for more than 8 hours with no sign of improvement.**

Headaches without fever

- Recurrent headaches not accompanied by fever have increased in the last few decades, particularly among children. They can mean many things and the cause must be determined by a doctor in each individual case. Please seek medical advice if you are concerned.
- Tension headaches

Symptoms

- Headache that proceeds primarily from the neck
- Stiff, tense neck muscles
- Dull pain or sensation of pressure in the forehead

How you can help

- Massage your child's neck with Aconit oil and keep it warm.
- School-age children can have a few drops of peppermint oil rubbed onto their temples. Don't use peppermint oil on infants, as there is a danger of choking.
- Do not give your child anything to eat. At most, they can have a few fat-free crackers and herb tea with a bit of lemon.
- Patience and rest will help ease the pain.

Migraines
Symptoms

- Cyclically recurring severe headaches, generally one-sided
- May begin with a so-called 'aura' (visual disturbances or other abnormal sensations)
- In some cases, sensitivity to sensory stimuli such as light, odours, noises
- Nausea and vomiting
- Abdominal symptoms may alone be present in children

How you can help

- Your child should sleep off a severe migraine attack in a quiet, darkened room.
- A cool compress of diluted arnica essence on the forehead and back of the neck may help (see page 309). Note that some children may be allergic to arnica.

Remedies

- Ferrum/Sulfur comp. globules, 5–7 globules 6 times a day.
- Wala Gentiana Stomach pellets, glob. velati, 5 globules up to hourly if nauseous.

The following constitutional treatments may be prescribed by your doctor:
- Weleda Kephalodoron (or Bidor) 0.1% or 5% tablets. Taking 2 tablets twice a day (before breakfast and lunch) for at least 3 months often reduces the frequency and severity of migraine attacks. Acute treatment with more frequent doses during an attack is perfectly safe.
- Additionally, Wala Gentiana Stomach pellets, glob. velati (5–7 globules before each meal).
- Alternatively, Secale/Quartz globules (5–7 globules 3 times a day).

Headaches while reading
Symptoms

- Recurring headache while reading
- Tired eyes or other vision problems

How you can help
- Visit an optometrist to check for nearsightedness, farsightedness or other vision problems.

General advice on headaches
- Regular sleeping habits and getting up at the same time each day are important. Do not allow your child to sleep in at the weekend.
- Make sure your child gets enough fresh air and physical activity.
- Limit time with TV, videos or computers, as these are potential triggers.
- 4 or 5 small meals are better than 3 large ones.
- Your child's regular diet should include easily digestible unsaturated fats, not too much protein, and plenty of vegetables and salads. In the morning, serve muesli or cereal; later on your child can have bread, fruit and yoghurt. Sweets (especially chocolate and fizzy drinks) should be limited.

- Pay attention to regular bowel movements, and treat flatulence as needed (see page 41).
- Aim for a regular, rhythmical daily and weekly schedule with regards to periods of both activity and rest (see page 244).
- Help your child keep a symptom diary for 4–8 weeks.
- Pay attention to possible interpersonal difficulties at home, in school and on other occasions. In some cases, consultation with an expert family therapist may be advisable.
- Do not underestimate the therapeutic potential of regulating, balancing activities such as curative eurythmy, music therapy or autogenic training.

2.2 Teething pains

General irritability and making pained noises when being laid down are usually signs of teething pain, earache or headache, because lying down increases the amount of blood in the venous vessels of the head. Fever is a possibility in all three cases and is almost invariably present in otitis media, which is an infection of the middle ear. Teething pain and earache can be confirmed through physical examination, but headaches can only be suspected when other causes have been eliminated (see page 27 for more on headaches). Teething pain can be ruled out if the mucous membrane covering the gums is uniformly pale in colour.

If teething pain is the culprit, note that doctors interested in their patients' overall development may find it important to know which tooth emerged at what age and whether anomalies of shape or location were present, so parents may find it useful to note this as children's teeth emerge. Teeth often erupt in the alphabetical order indicated schematically below:

GEFCBBCFEG

GEFDAADFEG

A and B are the central incisors, C and D the lateral incisors, F the canine teeth, and E and G the molars.

Symptoms
- Irritability
- Restlessness
- Expressions of pain when being laid down
- If molars are the cause of the symptoms, frequent rubbing of one ear (without other symptoms of otitis media, see page 33)
- Gums may be blood-darkened or swollen, with a tooth showing through
- In some cases, a slight temperature or even fever

How you can help
Remedies

- Giving your baby a piece of orris root to chew on can be helpful.
- Weleda Fever and Teething suppositories, 1–3 times daily, preferably at bedtime. These suppositories also have soothing, calming effects.
- Belladonna comp. suppositories for children, 1–3 times daily for teething accompanied by fever and restlessness.
- Nicotiana comp. glob. velati, 5 globules 3–6 times daily.
- In South Africa, Weleda Teething Remedy (Chamomilla/Millefolium comp.) drops are available.

2.3 Earache

Earache is common in children and is typically caused by an infection. It usually improves within a few days, but can be painful and distressing for your child.

Middle-ear infection (otitis media)

A more serious ear infection is otitis media, which involves redness and swelling in the middle ear and a build-up of fluid behind the eardrum. Many children experience this by time they are 10 years old, and the most commonly affected are infants. Take your child to your doctor to confirm the diagnosis. Infants who have been fully breast-fed for 3 months are less prone to middle-ear infections, while those who suck on dummies are more prone.

Straightforward otitis media only rarely requires antibiotic treatment. In our experience, myringotomy (puncturing the eardrum to draw off pus) is rarely necessary. If suitable means are used to help the body actively come to grips with the infection, the general strengthening that results means that relapses become less frequent.

Symptoms

- Tugging or rubbing the ear
- Slight hearing loss
- Loss of balance
- Irritability or restlessness
- Increased expressions of pain when being laid down
- Pained response to pressure on the tragus (the small, triangular projection just in front of the external opening of the ear).
- Signs of infections such as rhinitis and fever (see page 54)
- Later, discharge from the ear canal, occasionally pus
- Swelling and reddening behind the ear is an infrequent complication

How you can help

- Consult your doctor. Treating a middle ear infection is always a job for a medical professional.
- Hold a little pack of chopped onion or warmed dried chamomile flowers against the affected ear to offer pain relief (see page 294).
- Sea salt of 0.9% sodium chloride nasal spray or nose drops, initially hourly.
- As a preventative measure, ensure the feet are warm. In cold weather, a hat can help. Note that a headband may make things worse, as it leads to uneven distribution of warmth across the head.
- 3 or 4 weeks after getting better, see your doctor for a check-up.

General advice on ear care

When cleaning your child's ears, be careful to touch only the external ear and the visible part of the auditory canal with the swab. Deeper penetration disrupts self-cleaning of the auditory canal, which naturally moves old earwax away from the eardrum towards the outside.

If earwax becomes too dense, a daily drop of olive oil in the auditory canal (administered with your child lying on their side) is generally enough to soften it.

2.4 Eye pain: conjunctivitis

Causes

These are just some of the causes of conjunctivitis, of which there are many:

- Cold wind
- Allergies
- Infections
- Measles

Symptoms

- Reddening of the conjunctiva (the mucous membrane covering the white part of the eye and the inner surface of the eyelid)
- Persistent watery eye or suppurative secretion
- Sticky eyelids
- Avoidance of light
- The sensation of a foreign object in the eye, and (sometimes) itching
- **Severe pain is not typical of conjunctivitis and constitutes grounds for an immediate visit to the doctor or eye specialist**

How you can help

When treating eye irritation, it is important to distinguish between the following forms:

Inflammation with discharge in newborn babies involving one or both eyes needs treatment under doctor's supervision:

- Clean the lids with a sterile cotton swab and boiled water cooled to lukewarm (or better still, 0.9% sterile saline solution from a pharmacy). Because of the risk of allergic reactions and irritation from suspended particles, *do not* use chamomile tea.
- Then use Calendula 4X or Echinacea/Quartz comp. eye drops, 1 drop in each eye. Keep eye drops in the fridge and watch the expiry date.

Persistent watery eye is caused by blockage of the tear ducts draining into the nose. Droplets of pus often appear in the corners of the eyes closest to the nose.
- Sometimes carefully massaging the area of the nasal tear duct helps, using gentle pressure and a clean little finger.
- Echinacea/Quarz comp. eye drops, 1 drop in each eye, 3 times a day.
- An eye doctor can probe this delicate duct to clear it, but this measure is usually unnecessary.

Reddening and discharge in both eyes in the post-newborn stage accompanied by significant reddening of the conjunctiva and avoidance of light; eyelids tend to stick together.
- Clean the lids as described above for newborn babies.

- Calendula 4X or Echinacea/Quartz comp. eye drops, 3–4 drops in each eye once an hour to 'rinse out' the infection.
- If no improvement is noted in 2 or 3 days, take your child to the doctor.

Reddening and watering of both eyes, without discharge is usually due to sensitivity to wind, dust or smoke, or a symptom of hay fever.
- Euphrasia eye drops, 3–4 drops in each eye once an hour.
- In hay fever, Gencydo 0.1% or Echinacea/Quartz comp. eye drops, 1 drop in each eye, several times a day.

Reddening of one eye with or without discharge
- Caution is in order, since these symptoms may be due to either a foreign object in the eye or an inflammation of the cornea. It is best to go straight to the doctor.

2.5 Sore throat and neck pain

Sore throats and neck pains have many different causes. Sore throats are children's most common reason for refusing food. The appearance of the throat and the course of the illness vary, depending on the cause. Whenever pain is associated with refusing food, check first your child's stomach and then their mouth and throat. By pressing quickly and firmly on the back part of your child's tongue with a spoon handle or a tongue depressor, you can take advantage of the gag reflex to see your child's throat and tonsils. Just make sure to release the pressure quickly.

We have given symptoms and ways you can help for separate illnesses below.

Viral tonsillitis

Most cases of a sore throat are caused by viral tonsillitis. These infections are usually harmless.

Symptoms
- Glassy red spots (like fine grains of tapioca) along the gums
- Tonsils are somewhat red
- Tongue is coated
- A high fever (up to 40°C/104°F)
- May vomit

How you can help
- Apply cool throat wraps made with lemon juice or lemon slices to your child's throat (see page 296).
- Later, quark throat wraps may be appropriate (see page 297), especially when the lymph nodes of the throat are swollen.
- In milder cases, it's best to apply 'hot' lemon juice throat wraps (see page 296).
- Give your child sips of well-warmed sage tea with honey and lemon.
- Have your child gargle with a strong decoction of sage tea.
- Apply sweat packs (see page 312) in cases with only low-grade fever.
- Chemical disinfection of the mouth, as with mouthwash, is not useful.
- Use Echinacea mouth and throat spray or have your child gargle with Bolus Eucalypti comp. powder 3–5 times a day.
- For chronic or repeated tonsillitis, a 6–8 week course of mustard flour footbaths (see page 308) is helpful.
- Seek medical advice if you are concerned. Your doctor may prescribe stronger medications.
- Otherwise give Apis/Belladonna cum Mercurio, 5 globules 4–8 times a day.

Strep throat or septic sore throat

Usually, the bacteria responsible for strep throat or a septic sore throat are streptococci. Fortunately, the course of this disease is generally much milder now than it was in the past.

Possible complications include

middle-ear infections (see page 33), abscess formation around the tonsils, impetigo (see page 103) and (rarely) inflammation of the kidney (glomerulonephritis). Rheumatic fever (symptoms include acute polyarthritis and myocarditis) is a very infrequent complication (see also Scarlet fever, page 133).

For most doctors, the possibility of such severe complications constitutes grounds for insisting on the use of antibiotics and viewing any decision not to use them as an error in professional judgment. However, in some countries this is no longer recommended, as the excessive use of antibiotics leads to antibiotic resistance.

A point to consider, however, is that the sore throat that precedes the development of these rare streptococcal complications is often minor or even totally absent. Also, complications may occur in spite of early and thorough antibiotic treatment. (Reports from the US confirm that rheumatic complications can develop in spite of penicillin therapy.) In 10 years of treating strep throat, the one patient we saw who developed myocarditis had already received antibiotic therapy.

Furthermore, it has been shown that many people who are neither ill nor contagious have streptococci on their tonsils. For example, an experiment involving swabbing the throats of healthy kindergarten children showed that up to 30% of them had them. Given the fact that children have frequent contact with playmates, siblings and the many adults in their immediate surroundings, the possibility of streptococci recolonising the tonsils shortly after the conclusion of antibiotic treatment is high. It becomes obvious that even the widest possible use of penicillin cannot prevent the appearance of streptococcal complications with any degree of certainty.

We urge parents and doctors to arrive at mutually acceptable decisions for or against the use of antibiotics on a case-by-case basis. The majority of the patients we treated did not require antibiotics.

Symptoms
- Tonsils and the back of the gums are bright red, possibly spotted with white
- Other symptoms as for viral tonsillitis (previous page)
- **When the tonsils are thickly coated and bright red, a doctor should be consulted immediately to determine the cause, which may be glandular fever (infectious mononucleosis see Section 7.11). Diphtheria (Section 7.10) is a rare but possible cause of these symptoms.**

How you can help

- Seek medical advice, and maintain contact with your doctor every 2 or 3 days until your child is fever-free.
- Same as for viral tonsilitis (see page 36).
- Bed rest until at least 3 days after the fever abates.
- A check-up 2 or 3 weeks after symptoms have disappeared or at any point if your child's recovery progress is unsatisfactory.

Thrush

- See page 100 for fungus infection in the mouth.

Abscess on tonsils

Abscesses behind or under the tonsils rarely occur, but they are painful and require immediate medical attention.

Symptoms

- High, often fluctuating fever
- Feeling terrible
- Inability to open the mouth fully
- One-sided swelling displacing the uvula

How you can help

- **Take your child immediately to your nearest hospital Accident and Emergency department.** Tonsillar abscesses require prompt attention from a doctor, involving surgery and antibiotic treatment.

Lymph gland inflammation (Lymphadenitis)

Lymphadenitis takes one of two possible courses. Often, the swelling slowly recedes, although the lymph nodes may remain palpable for months as they gradually shrink. In other cases, parents will notice that the painful nodes grow noticeably bigger and harder each day. Ultimately, the skin covering the lymph node reddens and the lymph node adheres to it. These are signs that a lymph node abscess has developed. It will either rupture spontaneously or require lancing, in which case it leaves only a tiny scar.

In both cases, the body itself actively ensures that healing occurs. As a result, most children who have had such abscesses enjoy good resistance to suppurative infections for the rest of childhood. In our experience, therefore, it is worth avoiding antibiotic therapy while the illness is being overcome, although this must be decided with your doctor.

In almost every child, smaller lymph node swellings (swollen glands) can be detected during harmless infections or sometimes without any other sign of illness. Take your child to the doctor only if the painless swelling increases over several weeks.

Symptoms

- Lumpy, pressure-sensitive swelling (evident to the touch) on one or both sides of the neck below the jawbone
- Possible fever
- Note that swollen glands may occur with other throat complaints

How you can help

- It is safe to wait and observe how the illness progresses.
- Throat poultices with quark, eucaluptus or angelica (see page 295).
- Archangelica comp. Globules, 5–10 globules 3–6 times daily.

Myogelosis

Neck pain may also be caused by muscular contraction or inflammation of the lymph nodes located deep in the neck, or myogelosis. It is as painful as lumbago and has symptoms similar to meningitis (see page 27).

Symptoms

- Pain and hardening of the muscles at the back and side of the neck

How you can help

- Apply a warm oil compress, using either pure olive oil or 10% lavender oil, Wala Aconit pain killer oil or solum oil.

2.6 Chest pains

Painful breathing or coughing

Painful breathing or coughing usually means that the mucous membranes lining the airways are irritated (see also Croup page 72).

How you can help

- Steam inhalation with 0.9% solution of cooking salt.
- Honey-sweetened cough-relieving herbal teas.
- Warm oil compresses on the chest with 10% lavender or eucalyptus oils (see page 301). You can make either of these oils yourself by diluting the pure etheric oil with 9 parts of olive oil.

Pains in the chest wall

Pains in the chest wall occur when the muscles are irritated locally, rather like muscular rheumatism, during a respiratory infection or influenza.

Symptoms

- Sudden onset of sharp pain
- Trouble breathing deeply
- No cough
- May be mistaken for heart pains (although these are rare in childhood)

How you can help
- If you are concerned, seek medical advice immediately.
- Warm oil compress around the chest with 5–10% lavender or eucalyptus oils (see page 301).

Left-sided chest pain
Another type of chest pain is caused by accumulation of wind in the intestine under the left dome of the diaphragm.

Symptoms
- Trouble breathing deeply
- Between breaths there is a dull pressure on the left side of the chest, near the heart

How you can help
- If you are concerned, seek medical advice immediately.
- Caraway tea and other remedies known to relieve flatulence bring relief.
- Rubbing the area in a clockwise motion (make sure your hand is warm!) may also get the trapped wind moving.
- Sometimes the child can relieve the pain by pressing on their abdomen.

Pains originating in the heart
These are extremely unusual in children. Chest pains associated with a current or prior serious illness, racing pulse or curling up in the foetal position are signs that something is seriously wrong. Consult a doctor.

Pleurisy
Pleurisy is an inflammation of the tissue between the lungs and the ribcage. It is usually preceded by pneumonia.

Symptoms
- Pains in the ribcage
- High fever
- Jerky, interrupted exhalations

How you can help
- **Seek medical advice.** Pleurisy requires a visit to the doctor for a chest X-ray and possible hospitalisation for treatment.

Stitch in the side
A stitch in the side is usually caused by cramping of the lateral muscles of the abdominal wall and occurs while walking with a full stomach.

How you can help
- Instruct your child to hold their breath and press on their upper abdomen with their forearms while moving into a squatting position.

2.7 Abdominal pain

Various symptoms suggest abdominal pain, including cramps, crying, a stomach that feels tight or hard, pallor, a gurgling stomach, vomiting, lack of appetite and infrequent bowel movements. If you are concerned, go to see your doctor; however, it is possible for parents to perform some simple examinations themselves to distinguish harmless symptoms from dangerous ones and help their children feel better at home.

Flatulence (gas or wind)

Infants can often cry after a meal (although usually not while nursing). Possible causes include getting too much or too little to eat or drink, or they might not have managed to burp afterwards. Other than these circumstances, the most likely cause of the crying is either flatulence or strong intestinal peristalsis (the involuntary contraction of muscles that moves food through the digestive tract).

The classic 'cranky hour' in the late afternoon or evening has nothing to do with flatulence. For reasons that remain incompletely explained, infants often cry in the late afternoon or evening without seeming to be hungry or tired. Air swallowed while crying, however, may cause stomachaches.

Treatment is symptomatic and can range from patiently letting your baby 'cry it all out' through picking them up gently and massaging their feet to walking to and fro with them, calmly and rhythmically, perhaps humming quietly, until they fall asleep.

Not typical of wind pains are: vomiting (more than a couple of mouthfuls), a pale face, a tight abdomen, diarrhoea (multiple loose bowel movements between meals), failure to gain weight or sudden screaming indicative of intense pain. **Take your child to a doctor to determine the cause of these atypical symptoms.**

Symptoms
- Minor possetting (spitting up)
- Tight abdomen
- Straining to pass hard, normal or loose stools

How you can help
- Warmth is important: try a heated cloth or warm, moist abdominal compress made with chamomile, yarrow or lemon balm tea (see also page 304).
- Rub your baby's abdomen in a clockwise direction with a light massage oil (such as organic sunflower oil, olive oil or almond oil) infused with lemon balm or chamomile, or with 10% caraway oil, diluted 1:2 if needed.

- Dress your baby in wool under-shirts that cover the abdomen.
- Use warmer nappies.
- Put a warmed cherry-stone pillow on the abdomen.
- Keep your baby's knees warm too.
- Internally, a few spoonfuls of well-warmed fennel tea right before meals may help. Drops to relieve flatulence don't work any better than fennel tea.
- Carry your baby in a sling for 10 minutes after burping them.
- To soothe your baby after nursing, hold them on your upper thigh with their back to your chest and lightly massage their feet, ankles and calves (one foot with each hand). Letting a restless infant's kicking feet encounter the resistance of your hand is often enough to calm them.
- Monitor how much your child is eating (see page 192).
- Breastfeeding mothers could consider limiting consumption of wholegrain bread, raw rolled oats, hot spices, onions and cabbage, because this can make babies windy.
- Babies who are not breastfed may benefit from a change in formula, but **ask your doctor first** (see also page 195).
- In an infant, a cold can often be the cause of swallowing air. It can help to interrupt breastfeeding frequently and give your baby saline nose drops (0.9% NaCl) before you start.

Remedies

- Nicotiana comp. glob. velati, up to 3 globules per hour for cramp-like pains, otherwise 3 globules 3 times a day.
- Chamomilla Cupro culta, Radix Rh 3X, 5 drops before each feeding. These drops should be refrigerated.

Appendicitis

If you suspect appendicitis, seek medical advice. In toddlers, appendicitis may be difficult to recognise either because symptoms are mild or uncharacteristic, or because they immediately resemble acute abdominal disease (see page 45). Even for doctors, diagnosis is often not straightforward.

Symptoms

- Continuous, increasing pain that develops slowly over a period of hours and gradually becomes concentrated in the right lower abdomen
- Lack of energy
- Nausea
- Coated tongue
- Rejection of hot-water bottle
- Pain while walking and hopping

• In advanced stage, as in acute abdominal disease (page 45)

How you can help
• **Seek medical advice immediately.**
• Do not give your child anything to eat or drink.

Threadworms

Threadworms (oxyuris) are fragile, threadlike little creatures, 1–2 cm (½–1 in.) in length, that live in the rectum and lay their eggs outside the anus at night. The infection is transmitted to other children after scratching via fingernails and towels. The presence of eggs is easily confirmed by picking them off the unwashed anus in the morning with transparent tape, which is then stuck on a microscope slide for examination.

Symptoms
• Itching and sometimes eczema on the anus
• Possible abdominal pain at night
• Fine white threads may be visible in the stool

How you can help
• See remedies for Roundworms overleaf.

Roundworms

Roundworms (ascaris), which may cause abdominal pain, are much less common now than they once were. They are approximately 20 cm (8 in) long, but males are significantly smaller than females. They are transmitted on salads and other raw vegetables that have been fertilised with human excrement. The larvae develop inside the eggs for 30–40 days after ingestion. From the intestines, they travel by way of the portal vein, liver and heart to the lungs, where they break out of the pulmonary alveoli after about a week. Via the bronchi and the pharynx, they find their way back to the intestines, where they mature. Many different symptoms, including allergic reactions, may develop during this complicated journey. Worm eggs appear in the stools only after this developmental cycle is completed.

Symptoms
• Coughing, shortness of breath, bloody sputum
• Asthma symptoms may develop in children predisposed to allergies (see page 76 for asthma symptoms)
• Vomiting, nausea, abdominal pain
• Inflammation of the liver or bile ducts (infrequent)

How you can help
• You can help your child avoid relapses with careful hygiene

(washing hands with soap and a nail brush; no sharing of hand towels) and the following remedies.

Remedies

- Allium/Cuprum sulfuricum comp., 5–10 drops orally (depending on the age of the child), 3 times a day.
- Quartz 50% (less than 1/3 tsp. 3 times a day).
- Most parents today prefer a 1-day treatment of medicine prescribed by a doctor (several options are available). However, the above treatment prevents relapses.
- The success of the treatment is confirmed if microscopic clinical examination of a stool sample reveals no worm eggs after about 3 weeks.

Urinary tract infections

Urinary tract infections are common in children, but are usually not serious. However, consult your doctor to diagnose the particular problem quickly and to avoid it developing into something more serious, like a bladder infection.

A burning sensation while urinating is a common symptom, and sometimes it is so bad that your child may hold in their urine to avoid it. Note that the burning can disappear sooner than the infection, so it is sensible to have your child checked by a doctor to see if the infection is still present. Urine analysis is called for whenever such symptoms appear, although contamination or external infections in the genital area may produce false positives.

Serious kidney damage is possible when urinary tract infections occur frequently or become chronic. For this reason, **diagnosing and treating urinary tract infections is always a job for a doctor**.

Symptoms

- Abdominal or back pain (with or without fever)
- Pallor (i.e. unusual paleness of skin compared to your child's usual complexion)
- Generalised weakness
- Loss of appetite
- Wetting themselves or wetting the bed
- Burning sensation while urinating

How you can help

- Warm compresses with 10% eucalyptus oil over the bladder (see page 306).
- Keep your child's feet warm, rubbing them with solum oil as needed.
- Give your child plenty of warm drinks, such as herbal teas that include horsetail, *Solidago gigantea* (giant goldenrod), birch

leaves, restharrow root, nettle leaves, lemon balm and calendula flowers).

Remedies
• Cantharis Blasen glob. velati, 5 globules 4–8 times a day for irritable bladder.
• Berberis/Quartz glob. velati, 5 globules 4 times a day for irritable bladder.
• Argentum nitricum comp. glob. velati, 5–10 globules 3 times a day for at least 1 month for recurrent urinary tract infections.

Inguinal hernia
An inguinal hernia can appear as a swelling or bulge in your child's groin. It usually encloses part of the intestine. In girls it can enclose one of the ovaries, and in boys it can extend into the scrotum. It may be painful. Note that **any painful swelling in this part of the body requires prompt medical attention**.

Symptoms
• Bulging hernial sac, which can be any size, from as small as a nut to as large as an orange
• Possible pain in groin
• Possible difficulty passing stools

How you can help
• **Consult your doctor**: they may be able to push the contents of a hernial sac back into position.
• Inguinal hernias usually need surgery. (See also Hydrocele, page 51).

Acute abdominal disease
Constant severe abdominal pain accompanied by vomiting along with pallor and palpable abdominal changes (usually a painful tightening of the abdominal wall that makes it feel 'stiff as a board') are signs of acute abdominal disease, which can be life-threatening. **Seek medical help immediately.**

A hard abdomen can be a symptom of many different conditions, including a ruptured appendix, incarcerated hernia (bowel obstruction due to entrapment of the hernia's contents in the weak point of the abdominal wall), pancreatitis, kidney, gallstones etc. Parents who have not yet experienced the much less dangerous ketonic or acetonemic vomiting (see page 88) may confuse it with the symptoms of acute abdominal disease. Always consult your doctor if you are in doubt.

Sudden severe pain with no apparent cause, crying indicative of extreme pain, or vomiting that is not associated with a hard abdomen and showing sign of improvement within hours is reason to suspect intussusception (the slipping of a length of intestine into an adjacent portion).

Symptoms
- Constant severe abdominal pain
- Nausea and vomiting
- Pallor (i.e. unusual paleness of skin compared to your child's usual complexion)
- Generalised weakness
- Painful tightening of the abdominal wall that makes it feel stiff

How you can help
- **Call the emergency services or take your child to your nearest hospital Accident and Emergency department.** Your child needs immediate medical examination, ideally in hospital, where emergency surgery can be performed if necessary.

Abdominal pain with flu
Abdominal pain while having the flu can be very distressing for your child. However, the initial abdominal pain usually disappears once the typical sharp rise in fever occurs. This type of pain is distinct from appendicitis in that there is no localised sensitivity to pressure on the abdomen and the difference in temperatures measured rectally and under the arm is not more than 0.5°C/1°F. A fever that rises rapidly above 38.5°C/101.5°F is not typical of appendicitis.

Symptoms
- Abdominal pain in addition to flu symptoms (see page 66)
- Chills
- Lethargy, possible vomiting
- Headache and body aches

How you can help
- A hot-water bottle or warmed cherry-stone pillow on the abdomen feels good to a child with the flu, but is intolerable and dangerous to a child with appendicitis (see page 42).

Remedies
- Agrapyron glob. velati, 5 globules 3–6 times a day.

Abdominal pain associated with food intolerances
Food intolerances are on the rise even in early childhood. There are three distinct types:
- **Food allergies:** Frequent food allergens include milk, wheat, soy, nuts, egg, tomatoes, strawberries, citrus fruits and pork. In infants and toddlers, they often cause allergic eczema (see page 116) in addition to abdominal symptoms.
- **Food intolerances:** Lactose, fructose and sucrose intolerances are due to deficiencies in specific digestive aids, namely the enzymes that break down the sugars in question. Such deficiencies

may be genetically determined; for example, adults from Central and South Asia generally cannot digest lactose. These intolerances may also appear temporarily during periods of hormonal change, such as pregnancy or puberty, and they can also be triggered by gastrointestinal disorders such as inflammation, parasite infestation or allergies.

- **Coeliac disease:** This autoimmune disorder leads to gluten intolerance.

Symptoms

- Abdominal pain
- Flatulence
- Narrow or massive stools
- Eczema (in the case of food allergies)
- Nausea and vomiting and/or failure to thrive (in some instances)

How you can help

- Watch carefully to see if any of the above symptoms correspond to consumption of specific foods. Keeping a food diary for a period of time will make it easier for your child's doctor to diagnose the condition.
- Avoiding the food(s) in question is useful only after the doctor has clarified the situation, unless a certain food has obviously provoked an acute allergic reaction, in which case it should be avoided immediately (and possibly very strictly, depending on the severity of the reaction).

Remedies

- Cichorium e planta tota 5% glob. velati, 5 globules 3–6 times per day before meals, for narrow stools and eczema due to food intolerances.
- Wala Gentiana Stomach pellets, glob. velati, 3–5 globules before meals for at least 1 month, for food intolerances.

Other causes of abdominal pain

- Sore abdominal muscles caused by **overexertion** while playing or doing sports.
- Abdominal pain associated with **diarrhoea** (see page 85).
- When your young child complains of a stomachache, it is also worth checking their mouth for **inflamed tonsils** (see page 35). Children often interpret pain as coming from the stomach, or the pain may be due to the early stages of fever or to swollen abdominal lymph nodes.
- *Abdominal pains* may appear several hours to half a day before the onset of **acetonemic vomiting** (see page 88).
- Unusual thirst and increased urination for several days, with

or without abdominal pain, are signs of possible **diabetes mellitusn** (see page 155).

Psychosomatic abdominal pain

Psychosomatic means involving both the body and the mind. Children who complain of a stomachache often mean something else, such as, 'You haven't paid any attention to me today,' 'You're so busy working and it's no fun,' or 'I can't think of anything to do.'

Is your child 'pretending' to have a stomachache? Probably not. Children experience their surroundings with great intensity, so anything emotionally 'indigestible' that exceeds their level of tolerance can have immediate physical effects.

Stomachaches before or during school suggest **mental over-exertion** or **psychological stress factors** that should be discussed with your child's teacher. Your doctor may also be able to help explain the problem or suggest harmless helpful measures. As a rule, chemical sedatives or analgesics are not indicated.

We recommend reviewing your child's day with an eye to how you yourself may be contributing to the development of stomachaches. In many cases it is easy to recognise the cause and find a solution.

Sometimes it can be helpful to have an outsider help with this, e.g. a good friend, a teacher, the family doctor or even a child psychologist or psychiatrist.

Causes
- Birthday parties (too much excitement and overconsumption of cake).
- Experiencing outbursts of anger from a parent or teacher.
- Nervous anticipation or fear of failure before stage appearances, exams etc.
- Stressful family situations, such as conflicts, separations, deaths in the family, financial worries etc.
- Stress or overload experienced by a parent or teacher.
- Insufficient time for caregivers to surround the child with physical and psychological warmth and attention.
- The child's own ambition, jealousy etc.

How you can help
- Give your child positive reinforcement.
- Show warmth and take an interest in their day.
- Give them a sense of security, e.g. a structured daily schedule that includes rhythm, diversion, adequate rest and recreation.

In cases of stress at school

- Create a counterbalance to intellectual demands, e.g. by ensuring your child has time for friends, playing, sports or (as appropriate) relaxation exercises.
- Artistic activity, both active and passive, is helpful.
- Develop realistic plans for whether and how goals are to be achieved.
- Instead of pressuring your child to perform, try to stimulate their enthusiasm and interest.
- Ensure your child has support for learning disabilities, if applicable.
- Additional ideas can be found in the section on emotional pain (see page 167).

2.8 Musculoskeletal pain

The causes and manifestations of this type of pain are so variable that few generalisations are possible. Regardless of whether an accident has occurred or the pain appears spontaneously, it is essential for parents to attempt to get as complete a picture as possible of what led up to the pain. Is there any new or temporary swelling or unusual warmth in the painful area? It is helpful for the doctor to know about these signs and when they first appeared, as well as any signs of fever. They may indicate serious underlying illnesses, such as rheumatic disorders, osteomyelitis (an inflammatory bone disease) and other diseases that we will not discuss here. Fortunately, they are rather uncommon. In any case, they always require thorough medical investigation.

Limping in toddlers

A child who is in pain will naturally avoid any movement that exacerbates it. Before consulting your doctor, examine the soles of your child's feet. You may find a callus, a spot where a shoe pinches or an injury from stepping on a tack or the like.

Be aware that if a family member or acquaintance limps, your child may be copying this behaviour. Muscle soreness after unaccustomed exertion can also cause limping.

Finally, inflammatory irritation of the hip joints ('irritable hip' or 'transient synovitis') can occur during or shortly after infections. Such irritation is usually short-lived. Medications to relieve inflammation include:

Remedies

- Rhus toxicodendron comp., 5 globules 3–6 times per day.
- Stannum metallicum 0.4% ointment, thinly applied to the painful inguinal area 2 times per day.

- **Seek medical advice once you are sure that the limp does not have a harmless cause.**

Contusions, strains, sprains

In the case of a bad fall or accident, your child should be seen by a doctor to ensure there are no torn ligaments or bone fractures. Medications to relieve inflammation include:

Remedies

- Arnica or calendula compresses or ointments (see page 309) (note that some children may be allergic to arnica).
- Arnica e planta tota 3X or 6X glob. velati, 5–10 globules 4 times a day.

2.9 Phimosis, hydrocele, undescended testicle

These conditions involving the male genitals seldom cause pain, but we will cover them here because they sometimes require surgical intervention. With or without phimosis, occasional erections may occur, beginning in infancy. Little boys sometimes report pain or a sensation of tightness associated with their erections. Juvenile erections are not a sign that your child is masturbating. They are especially likely to occur during sleep, in the early morning hours.

Phimosis (constriction of the foreskin)
Symptoms

- Foreskin will not slide over the glans
- Sometimes the foreskin sticks to the glans

Complications

- Accumulation of smegma (a white, crumbly deposit of cast-off epithelial cells that accumulate between the foreskin and the glans).
- Painful inflammation of the foreskin (balanitis).
- Scar tissue (which may may develop as a result of improper stretching of the foreskin), chronic irritation or inflammation.
- Urinary retention (possible but uncommon).

How you can help

- In most cases the best approach is initially to do nothing, as the problem may sort itself out. Most boys outgrow phimosis by age 2, but 8% of boys ages 5–6 and roughly 1% of those ages 16–18 still have phimosis that requires treatment. We recommend routine cleaning of the glans only after onset of puberty or when significant amounts of smegma develop. Before that, external cleansing is sufficient.

In case of prolonged
constriction or adhesion

- Careful moving of the foreskin in a warm bath.
- Apply Rosatum Heilsalbe cream 2 times per day.
- Doctors may prescribe treatment with oestrogen or cortisone creams, they may free the foreskin with a bulb-headed probe, or shorten the foreskin (circumcision) under suitable anesthesia.

Hydrocele

A hydrocele is a swelling in the scrotum that occurs when fluid accumulates around a testicle. When the gonads descend before birth from the abdominal cavity through the inguinal canal into the scrotum, they pull the peritoneum (the smooth lining of the inside of the abdominal cavity) with them. Before this projection of the peritoneum closes completely, blister-like remnants may persist and may be filled with fluid when irritation occurs. Hydroceles usually disappear spontaneously in infancy.

Symptoms

- Swollen scrotum

How you can help

- Don't press on them while putting a nappy on your baby.

- If hydroceles persist in preschool boys, surgery is often performed, especially if an inguinal hernia also requires correction.

Undescended testicle

An undescended testicle is diagnosed when no testicle is evident in the palpated scrotum. (A retractile testicle descends when a child is sitting in a warm bath and retracts again in colder conditions. Retractile testicles do not require surgical intervention.) Undescended testicles require surgery and you should consult your doctor.

The optimal age for undergoing the surgical procedure has not yet been agreed upon universally, but current guidelines recommend having it done before age 1 to avoid any risk of reduced fertility. On the other hand, from the point of view of anthroposophic medicine, early surgical intervention is an assault on the fabric of the child's body and soul and may have a variety of consequences. For this reason, it is essential to confirm that the child's mother or father can accompany him to the clinic. In individual cases, it is certainly acceptable to consider a later date.

Before resorting to the surgical procedure, many paediatricians and surgeons recommend hormonal treatment, which usually consists of GnRH nasal spray for younger boys and the addition of HCG injections for older ones. This hormone treatment, because it stimulates the reproductive organs in a way similar to their natural stimulation in pre-puberty, also induces psychological shifts that may include aggressive personality changes. Any hoped-for improvement in later fertility has not yet been adequately confirmed, and in fact early hormone treatment has been shown to cause sperm cell damage in a small number of cases.

While hormone treatment does promote testicular descent (at least in the absence of mechanical obstructions), the descent is often not permanent and the need for surgery is not eliminated. Loosening of the tissues also occurs, which some surgeons view as desirable because it makes surgery easier, should it prove necessary. In most cases, the little boy's penis becomes somewhat larger and does not return to its original size when treatment is stopped.

We do not recommend hormone treatment. It disrupts a child's hormone levels unnecessarily and has adverse effects on their physical and emotional make-up.

Symptoms
- No testicle is evident in the palpated scrotum
- It may be possible to feel the testicle in the groin

How you can help
- Before resorting to a surgical procedure, we recommend at least 2 months of constitutional treatment, (see page 248), prescribed by your doctor, which may include some of the following remedies.

Remedies
- Argentum metallicum prep. 6X trituration, 1 pea-sized portion 3 times a day, supplemented with an external application of:
- Argentum metalicum prep. 0.4% ointment to the groin at bedtime, and:
- Epiphysis/Plumbum glob. velati, 5 globules in the morning and in the evening, alternating weekly with:
- Hypophysis/Stannum glob. velati, 5 globules in the morning and in the evening.
- We do not recommend attempting hormone therapy (see previous page).

3. Fever and its Treatment

Fever is a decisive aid to processing and overcoming the bodily challenges that occur during many illnesses. Other functions and activities, such as eating, digestion, sensory perception, interest in one's surroundings, play and so forth, take second place to the body's efforts to produce a fever. In this chapter we will discuss the causes of fever before describing some typical fevers that your child may experience and giving advice on how to treat them at home.

3.1 What causes fever?

In children, fever is most often caused by inflammatory illnesses: usually harmless influenzas, respiratory, throat or ear infections. **Recognising serious infections is a matter of experience and requires medical attention.**

Elevated body temperature can occur due to overheating when the body cannot give off enough heat to compensate for excess heat entering from outside, for instance when sleeping under a blanket in a heated room or sleeping in a car when the sun is shining. It can occur with an infant sleeping in their parents' bed (see page 223). In infants, this type of temperature quickly disappears when the cause (blanket, bonnet or leggings) is removed.

Dehydration can also cause a fever, particularly with diarrhoea and vomiting (see page 85). Make sure your child has enough to drink. Take care when giving drinks to a child who is vomiting that they do not immediately afterwards vomit again and get into a vicious circle (see Vomiting and diarrhoea, page 86). Encourage them to drink very slowly, keeping a sip in their mouth for a time before taking the next one.

Vigorous movement can also cause body temperature to rise above 38°C/100.5°F. In such cases, check again after your baby or child has been lying still for half an hour.

3.2 Taking your child's temperature

We recommend using high-quality digital thermometers, which are quick and reliable. Ear thermometers still vary greatly in quality and are especially unreliable in the case of ear infections. Most infrared thermometers, temple thermometers and forehead thermometer strips are too inaccurate.

- Temperatures up to 37.5°C/ 99.5°F are considered normal.
- A temperature between 37.5°C and 38°C (99.5°F and (100.5°F) is elevated but subfebrile (i.e. not feverish).
- A temperature of 38°C/ 100.5°F or higher is considered a fever.
- For an infant under 3 months with a fever over 38 °C who is not drinking or looks unwell, seek medical help immediately.
- Most children can tolerate a high fever, but if your child is feeling unwell and you are concerned, seek medical help.

3.3 Signs of fever and treating fevers

If your child seems different or you think they look unwell, more detailed observation is in order. Is your child moving the way they normally do? Is their tongue dry? Have they got dark rings around their eyes? Check their eyes, nostrils and breathing; feel the warmth of their forehead, neck, torso and limbs. Touch their abdomen and note any signs of pain. Take their temperature as just described. If you are unfamiliar with or concerned about the symptoms you observe, call your doctor.

Your own experience and confidence in assessing feverish conditions is paramount, so if you are uncertain, consult your doctor. One of the most gratifying experiences for a doctor is to see how parents develop confidence over time and have less and less need of their advice.

Rising fever

The body develops the heat of a fever through increased metabolic activity in all the muscles in the body and reduced blood supply to the skin.

Symptoms during rising fever
- Pale skin colour (pallor)

- Cool limbs
- Chills
- Restlessness
- Discomfort, possibly with head-ache
- Aching limbs
- Abdominal pain
- Vomiting

How you can help
- During a rising fever, the body cannot yet give off excess heat. *Do not*, **under any circumstances, apply cool compresses to your child's calves during this initial stage**, as calves and feet only start getting hot after the fever has peaked.
- Keep your child's surroundings quiet and peaceful.
- Keep your child's wrists and ankles warm by applying a warmed cherry-stone pillow and rubbing in some solum oil.
- Give warm herb tea, such as lemon balm, slightly sweetened if necessary.
- Food is not necessary at this stage, particularly as your child may feel nauseous.

Remedies
- Warm compresses on the wrists made with arnica essence (see page 309). (Note that some children may be allergic to arnica.)
- Infludoron, 5 globules every hour or two until about 4:00 pm

(later it may prevent children from sleeping).
- Aconitum/China comp. suppos-itories may help.

Fever peak
In the next phase, the fever rises to the level the body is attempting to achieve.

Symptoms
- Red cheeks
- Sparkling eyes
- Hot head
- Warm hands and feet
- Weakness, fatigue
- Hallucinations (in some cases)

How you can help
- A restless child may refuse to stay covered and want to get up and run around in spite of a fever. They need the calming presence of an adult who will sing, hum, tell stories or engage in some other quiet activity. For younger children, it's useful to have a portable cot that you can move around the house so your child can accompany you as you work. Older children might like to spend the day on a sofa in the living room. Provide simple toys that leave room for the imagination (see page 221).
- Give your child light clothing and bedding.

- Ensure there is fresh air in the room, but no draughts.
- Give your child plenty of fluids: for instance, cool or lukewarm diluted fruit juice (cherry, blackcurrant, pear or lemon; Weleda Blackthorn Elixir).
- Stick to a bland diet with no potatoes and little fat or protein: no nuts, chocolate etc. Do not try to maintain weight in a child with a fever; they will quickly gain it back after the illness is over.
- If your child's skin feels hot all the way to the calves, apply leg compresses if their temperature is over 39°C/102°F (see page 307). Cool sponging can also be used. This is especially good with headaches induced by the fever. These measures support the body's efforts to eliminate excess heat through the skin, but only apply them if they feel comfortable to your child.
- Generally this will keep your child's temperature between 39°C and 40°C (102°F–104°F), which can be tolerated by most children. It is better to keep the temperature at a certain level than induce strong variations, as this puts a strain on the circulation.

Remedies

- For a very high fever, give Apis/Belladonna glob. velati, 5 globules up to half-hourly.

- Weleda Fever and Teething suppositories or Heel Viburcol, at most every 6 hours in the acute phase.

Fever suppressants (ibuprofen or paracetamol/acetaminophen)

Generally, such fever suppressants impair the immune system. It is better to hold the fever at the level the body needs than to lower the fever, which causes temperature differences that strain the circulation.

In rare cases, if your child suffers from pain or is generally feeling unwell and the above measures have not worked, you can administer an age-appropriate dose of ibuprofen (Advil or Motrin) or paracetamol/acetaminophen. However, **consult your doctor**.

It is no longer recommended to take fever suppressants to prevent febrile seizures, as these tend to take place during a sudden rise in temperature rather than during the longer fever peak.

Fever reduction and convalescence

Once the fever has served its purpose, the body begins to reduce it. The release of heat is apparent all over the body.

Symptoms

- Reddened cheeks grow pale
- Sweating
- Exhaustion that may still persist

How you can help

- For heavy sweating, give 1 cup of sage tea in the morning.
- Ensure that your child stays warm enough. Premature exposure to cold or dampness can lead to relapse.
- Ensure that your child stays quiet for long enough before cautiously resuming their normal activities.

Remedies

- Meteoric iron, glob. velati or rose iron, glob. velati, 5–10 globules 3 times a day for approximately 4 weeks.

When to seek medical help

- For an infant under 3 months with a fever over 38°C who is not drinking or looks unwell, contact your doctor immediately.
- If your baby has a febrile convulsion or seizure (see Section 3.4).
- For any fever that significantly impacts your child's state of health, e.g., is accompanied by significant drowsiness, headache, stiff neck, other diffuse or severe pains, significantly laboured breathing, considerable fluid loss through diarrhoea or vomiting, or if your baby does not want to drink anything.
- The fever rises above 40°C but your baby's skin still feels cool.
- Any fever that varies up and down by more than 1.5°C (without chemical fever-reducing medication).
- Your child continues to seem severely affected in spite of effective fever-reducing measures.

3.4 Febrile seizures

Febrile seizures, or febrile convulsions, are fits that can occur when your child has a fever. **A child's first incident of seizure-like loss of consciousness, with or without convulsions, is always reason to call your doctor. If the seizure continues, take your child to your doctor or to your nearest hospital Accident and Emergency department as quickly as possible** (see also Fainting and Breath-holding attacks, page 18 and page 19).

Febrile seizures are of two types: simple and complex. A simple febrile seizure is isolated and brief (lasting less than 15 minutes). The majority of febrile seizures are simple febrile seizures. Complex febrile seizures last for more than 15 minutes, may be multiple (i.e. more than one seizure occurs) and the seizure occurs in a single area of the brain (symptoms may begin as a stare, or jerking on one side of the body).

Febrile seizures are common in the first few years of life (2–5% of children have them between the ages of 6 months and 5 years). The immature brain has a lower convulsion threshold than the adult brain: i.e. it reacts to elevated temperatures with much greater sensitivity.

About a third of children who have febrile seizures may have a further seizure. Only 2 out of every 100 children who have febrile seizures go on to develop a convulsive disorder.

By themselves, febrile seizures do not cause lasting damage or behavioural or developmental disorders, and neither are they associated with sudden infant death (SIDS). Febrile seizures do not 'cause' epilepsy, although they may be the first sign of it in children predisposed to convulsions. The risk of developing epilepsy increases only with repeated fever convulsions (more than 4), a family history of epilepsy or complex febrile seizures.

Simple febrile seizure
Symptoms
- Bilaterally symmetrical rhythmical twitching of the extremities
- Stiffening of the whole body
- Rising fever
- Lasts less than 15 minutes
- Occurs between ages or 1 and 5

How you can help
- Stay calm.
- Note how long the seizure lasts.
- Do not hold your child tight and do not place anything between their teeth.
- If your child is in danger of choking, lay them securely on their side.
- Consult your child's doctor.

Precautionary measures
- Make sure that your child is dressed warmly enough to avoid precipitating or exacerbating the initial chill stage of the fever when the feet and calves are cold and need warming.
- When their head becomes sweaty, cool the forehead and temples with a wet washcloth.
- Avoid worrying or exciting a child with a high fever.
- Avoid background noise and media.
- Fever suppressants (ibuprofen or paracetamol/acetaminophen) cannot prevent febrile seizures nor stop the development of a lasting seizure disorder.

Remedies
- Belladonna Rh 6X dilution: during initial stage of fever 5 drops every 15 minutes or put

20 drops into a cup of herb tea to be sipped over the course of an hour; during high fever 5 drops every half hour.

- Belladonna comp. child suppositories, maximum every 6 hours.
- Your doctor may prescribe appropriate constitutional remedies (anthroposophic or homeopathic) to address any imbalances in the body's reactive status.

Complex febrile seizures
Symptoms
- Symptoms are one-sided or begin in one place
- The seizure lasts more than 15 minutes
- The seizure recurs within 24 hours
- The seizure occurs outside the typical age range of 1–5

How you can help
- If your child has already been prescribed with diazepam rectal suppositories by a doctor, administer one immediately.
- If the seizure has not stopped after 3 minutes, call for emergency medical assistance or immediately take your child to your nearest hospital Accident and Emergency department.
- Seizures of this type require further diagnostic testing, such as an EEG.

3.5 The purpose of fever

Fever is a crisis-like change in the body's warmth system. Its causes are varied. For a child, even a birthday party, a long trip, a sudden change in the weather, overcooling or an erupting tooth may overburden the body, leaving it susceptible to colonisation by germs.

Animal experiments have shown that viruses and bacteria reproduce best and are thus most likely to cause damage at temperatures of 33–35°C/91–95°F: that is, below normal body temperatures. Hence the expression 'to catch cold' is quite apt. On the other hand, fevers provide optimum temperatures (generally 39–40°C/102–104°F) for killing or preventing the proliferation of the viruses or bacteria that affect the body.

Fever stimulates the activity of the immune system, preventing the proliferation of viruses or bacteria. Fever suppression with measles can lead to complications and with an unrecognised 'blood poisoning' (lymphangitis) where bacteria multiply in the blood, affecting the organs. Fever suppressants also lower the efficacy of the kidneys. An international study of over 200,000 children from 31 countries has even demonstrated that administering paracetamol/acetaminophen before age 1 is associated with a significant increase in cases of bronchial asthma in 5- to 6-year-olds.

Research has shown that fevers in early childhood prevent allergies. The risk of cancer is lowered, particularly after measles, mumps, German measles and chickenpox.

Not only fever suppressants but also antibiotics can interrupt the body's activities and should therefore be administered only when the body cannot hold its own against a bacterial infection. And in any case, antibiotics are ineffective against viruses, which are implicated in more infections than bacteria.

Fever is a highly effective reaction of the body to combat illness and lay the foundation for sound health.

Thermoregulation and fever also have a soul-spiritual aspect. Heat is more than just a quantitative factor measured with a thermometer; warmth also manifests in the activity of the human soul and spirit. We 'feel warm inside' when we meet a good friend or revisit the familiar landscape of our childhood. When we have a good idea or wax enthusiastic about an ideal, warmth can literally shoot into our limbs. Conversely, fear, anger or great sorrow, or even hate, envy or discontent in our surroundings, makes our 'blood run cold'. We may speak of an icy mood, frosty silence or a cold refusal, or we may say, 'That leaves me cold.'

Just as a comfortable body temperature of 37°C/98.5°F supports the activities of body, soul and spirit, so too a joyful experience, inner concentration or meditative work can have harmonising effects on how the body is pervaded with warmth. Blood circulation and the supply of blood to the organs are sensitive not only to the body's movement and nutrition but also to our emotions and thoughts. We quite rightly relate warmth to the soul and spirit as well as to the body. At all three levels, the same warmth is at work, although it is sometimes more inwardly and sometimes more outwardly active.

The unified nature of warmth allows us to experience ourselves as self-contained physical and soul-spiritual beings. Hence we can say that the body's warmth organisation as a whole is the physical vehicle of the self, the human 'I'. Every illness is accompanied by a change in this warmth system and thus affects and involves the 'I' in a very direct way.

We owe thanks to Rudolf Steiner's research into the human constitution for recognising this connection and making it bear fruit in education and medicine. We change our attitude towards illness when we see it as related to a child's own activity and volition that is, to his or her 'I'. Hence the individual differences the child who 'never' runs a fever, the one whose fevers remain slight and rise slowly, the one who gets brief attacks of high fever. We meet whole families of children who are always the first to be flat on their backs while the neighbour's kids are still splashing in the puddles. Then they switch roles, and the last one to catch cold may have the longest struggle with the infection.

Other individual differences become evident in adults. A person who enjoys their work and works long and hard but rhythmically may be much less susceptible to colds and flu than someone who takes a lot of time off to 'relax'. When we enjoy our work, when the 'I' is heavily involved in it, our warmth system is stimulated, 'immunising' us against illness. Psychoneuroimmunological research has confirmed that positive emotions like courage, enthusiasm, trust and love stimulate the human immune system, while stress, anger, fear, lethargy and depression weaken it.

Hence, when we confront the high fevers of childhood infectious diseases, we must ask about the purpose of each fever. Is it an attempt to temporarily strengthen the soul-spiritual element's ability to intervene in the body? Or is it meant to create a substitute for a lack of soul activity? We can make many interesting observations that help to answer these questions.

Here is a very telling example. Relatives who initially say a new-born baby 'looks just like their grandfather' may later change their minds and decide that they look more like their mother. But after the baby undergoes a feverish illness, the parents discover a new trait not found among their relatives and are pleased to see their child's own unique personality emerging. Fever helps a child's 'I' adapt its inherited body to its own purposes, making it a more suitable vehicle for self-expression.

Predisposition to diseases such as eczema or asthma in infancy has been known to improve after serious feverish illnesses. A possible physiological explanation for this phenomenon, as suggested by the immunological and genetic research of the last decades, is that a person's genetic material is not a fixed entity, as was previously assumed, but rather a dynamic one that may manifest differently under different circumstances.

It has long been known that genes and their functions are influenced not only by the immune system but also by soul-spiritual and psycho-social processes throughout the person's lifetime.

From a purely outer perspective, the rapid regaining of weight lost during a feverish illness is an indication that the body is being organically remodelled. The child has deconstructed some aspect of their inherited body and is rebuilding it under the independent direction of their own warmth organisation. In our own paediatric practices, we have experienced repeatedly that flu with a high fever, a carefully managed case of pneumonia or even measles may introduce a new, more stable phase in a child's development. Less frequently, longer bouts of repeated illness indicate a task that remains to be accomplished.

Fever's effect on the body can be compared to good educational methods under both circumstances, the child learns something through their own efforts. Constantly telling children 'Do this; don't do that; you're not allowed to do that' is generally considered poor educational practice. Unfortunately, this is exactly what happens in many feverish infections. As soon as a child's temperature exceeds 38.5°C/101.5°F, they are given fever-suppressing medication, and if infection is confirmed antibiotics are prescribed too, leaving the body with little chance for independent involvement. Furthermore, a body thus treated loses an opportunity to practise the 'flexibility' it will need to confront tasks more serious and more important than overcoming the feverish infections of childhood.

Of course we know that dramatic and extreme reactions such as febrile seizures can occur and that with some infectious diseases permanent damage is possible. Complications, although infrequent, must be caught in time, so it is important to be alert and cautious around childhood feverish illnesses. If in doubt always seek medical help.

4. Respiratory Diseases

Respiratory obstruction is a common cause of visits to the paediatrician. Good, lasting treatment targets not only the directly affected lungs but also your child's whole body and emotional state. This is especially true of treatment for chronic disorders such as bronchial asthma or recurrent bronchitis. In these very common childhood illnesses, it is especially important to include valuable therapeutic approaches that also consider the acute problem in the context of nutrition, digestion, thermal regulation and adequate physical activity. Below, we discuss common respiratory ailments in childhood.

In contrast to conventional medical treatment, anthroposophic treatment of patients with acute respiratory or ear symptoms achieves a milder course of the illness, significantly lower prescription rates for antibiotics and fewer drug side effects, all with higher patient satisfaction.

4.1 Nasal congestion

Be ready to nip it in the bud. A simple case of the sniffles might seem harmless and safe to ignore, but it is a typical early symptom of almost all infections in the respiratory passages and ears. Therefore taking note of nasal congestion can help with early detection, prevention and treatment.

Nasal congestion in very young infants is not harmless and must be monitored and treated by a doctor. In the first 3–4 weeks of life, a baby has not yet learned to breathe through their mouth, so when their nose is blocked they get air only when they cry. Nasal blockage can cause a serious oxygen shortage, up to and including cyanosis (turning blue).

Sniffling and snoring sometimes persist for months after an infant's first cold but will disappear in time. No treatment is needed as long as your baby can breathe freely. It will pass in time.

Sneezing removes bits of solid matter from the nose. In infants, it generally does not indicate the beginning of a cold. Crusts in a baby's nose are more likely to be caused by regurgitated milk or by dry, heated air than by inflamed mucous membranes.

For older children, the use of decongestant drops or sprays is questionable. Nasal discharge serves a purpose; a cold is a self-limiting condition that should be allowed to run its course unhindered. Decongestants constrict the blood vessels of the mucous membranes; the alternation between this constriction and subsequent dilation when the medication wears off disrupts the natural course of healing. Frequent use can also dry out and damage the nasal mucous membranes, which in turn may eventually lead to ozaena, a chronic nasal disease characterised by foetid discharge and atrophic structural changes.

Often multiple causes and symptoms are present simultaneously. For example, irritation due to allergies or cold weather paves the way for pathogens, so recurrent respiratory infections are common in winter (and especially typical) in children with dust mite allergies.

Causes
• Allergies (secretions are usually clear and fluid)
• Dust (nasal secretions are clear and contain particles of dirt)
• Viruses (secretions are fluid and clear to whitish)
• Bacteria (secretions are yellow to greenish, stringy and slimy to crusty)
• Chemical or mechanical irritation (uncommon)

Symptoms
• Obstructed nasal breathing
• Difficulty in drinking and signs of respiratory distress are possible in infants
• Swollen and red nasal mucosa
• Nasal secretions are clear to yellow-green, and can be anything from fluid to dry and crusty
• Nostrils may be reddened

How you can help
For infants
• Make sure the room has fresh, moist air. Hang damp cloths in the room, rewetting them frequently, possibly adding a little lavender bath milk.
• Air the room, but in cool weather your baby should be warmly dressed in soft wool and well covered, especially the head and ears.
• Only water-based medications or breast milk should be applied to the mucous membranes inside the nose. Smear a drop of breast milk into the infant's nose. This not only provides moisture but

also immune active substances (antibodies).

- A 1% sodium chloride solution (physiological saline), carefully inserted into the nose one drop at a time, is often the only medication needed. You can buy this solution in your pharmacy or make it at home by adding 1 teaspoon of table salt (about 4.5 grams) to ½ litre (US 2 cups) of water. Bring the solution to the boil and then pour some of it into a clean glass jar. It keeps for about 2 days, but sterilise the dropper in boiling water once a day.
- Decongestant nose drops are sometimes avoidable, but if you must use them, make sure that the brand is intended for use in infants and does not contain ephedrine, and never use the drops for more than a few days.

For older children

- Inhale steam from chamomile tea (see page 312).
- Nasal irrigation: rinse with a lukewarm 2% salt solution (approximately 2 g table salt in 100 ml boiled water, or 1 teaspoon per US cup). Sniff up the liquid out of a cup through the nose and spit it out through the mouth. Since the concentration of salt is higher in the solution than it is in nasal discharge, this treatment is a natural means of reducing swelling in the mucous membranes and clearing the entrances to the paranasal sinuses. This procedure, although not exactly pleasant, is extremely effective.

- If your child has dry, red mucous membranes at the entrance to their nose, apply a specially formulated nasal cream available from your pharmacy (e.g. nasal balsam, angelica balsam or marjoram cream).

Remedies

- Berberis/Quarz glob. velati, 5 globules 3–6 times a day if the mucus is clear and flowing.
- Sambucus comp. glob. velati, 5 globules 3–6 times a day if the mucus is green and infected.
- Silicea comp. glob. velati, 5 globules 3–6 times a day for a cold with fever or for children prone to ear infections.

Preventative measures

- Pay attention to warmth. In particular, keep your child's head, ears and feet warm. The common 'cold' needs to be taken literally!
- Make sure your child gets enough fresh air and exercise.
- For children allergic to dust mites, we recommend long-term use of the nasal irrigation procedure described above.

4.2 Viral infections: colds and flu

A cold as described in Nasal congestion (page 63) is often a first sign of a viral infection. Often no distinction is clear between a 'cold' and a 'flu' (influenza), but an illness that begins with headaches and body aches is generally called flu. A respiratory infection may be accompanied by inflammation and discharge in the air cavities of the skull, which include the ethmoid, maxillary and frontal sinuses (note that the frontal sinuses do not develop until children are of school age). Inflammation occasionally also occurs in the middle ear (see page 33) and in the petrosal bone that surrounds the inner ear.

The pharynx and its 'lymphatic apparatus' are always involved, namely the tonsils at the back of the mouth as well as the lymphatic tissues at the sides and back of the throat. These lymphatic organs are most important points in the interplay between the body and its environment.

True cases of influenza (not to be confused with Haemophilus influenzae type B or Hib infections; see Section 14.5) are difficult to recognise among the many viral infections of childhood, although they are sometimes distinguished by their slightly greater severity (see also flu vaccinations page 280, Section 14.20).

Children who are well cared for generally recover spontaneously from the great majority of flu-type infections within a few days and without developing complications. Symptom-suppressing treatments such as fever reducers, cough suppressors, decongestants and antibiotics to prevent bacterial infection simply impose additional, unnecessary burdens on the body. A child who is otherwise healthy will overcome such infections without help and acquire at least temporary immunity (see also Section 14). However, we understand that parents want to make their children more comfortable while the illness is taking its course, so you may find the measures below helpful.

Symptoms

- Nasal congestion
- Sore throat
- Possibly coughing or hoarseness are typical of a cold
- Headache and aching limbs are typical of flu
- Fever
- Sinusitis that becomes more painful on leaning forwards
- Rhinitis (inflammation of the mucous membranes of the nose.

Seek medical advice if:

- Your child has a fever over 38.5°C/101.5°F that lasts for more than 3 days. This suggests that the original infection has paved the way for a more serious illness.
- Your child has a persistent, troublesome cough that appears to affect the lower respiratory tract.

How you can help

- Encourage your child to drink a lot.
- A sick child should avoid excitement and be allowed to sleep a lot.
- A little doll or a gnome who peeks out from under the covers or climbs pillow mountains will provide hours of amusement.
- Provide fresh air that is not too dry. If necessary, use a vaporiser or hang damp cloths in the room.
- Spread a little eucalyptus oil, Olbas oil or Babix Inhalat on a cloth or saucer and set it on a heat source in the room (not in the bed, and not for children who have asthma, see page 76).
- For nasal congestion see Section 4.1.
- If your child is coughing, rub their chest with 10% lavender or mallow oil. Alternatively, use chest rubs (see page 302) with or without hot, moist compresses.
- If your child is shivering, keep them warmly covered. If needed, give your child hot tea to drink and pile on extra covers to induce sweating. Afterwards, change them into dry bedclothes.

Remedies

- Gelsemium comp. glob. velati, 5 globules every half hour for flu with headache.
- Weleda Infludoron; formerly available under the name Ferrum phosphoricum comp.), up to 5 globules per hour at the beginning of a cold. Stop giving these globules in the evening because they can cause wakefulness, increasing the likelihood of coughs and asthma.
- Angocin, 1–2 tablets 3 times daily for sinus involvement.
- For coughs, thyme tea with honey or the following cough syrups are good: Weleda Lichen-Honey syrup, Weleda cough elixir and Wala Pulmonium cough liquid.
- For rhinitis accompanied by a sinus infection, you can rub the areas of the frontal and maxillary sinuses with Cochlearia armoracia 10% ointment.

Preventative measures

- In addition to the suggestions in Section 4.1, Nasal congestion, Echinacea syrup can be used to stimulate the body's own healing forces. The dosage is ½–1 teaspoon, 3 times a day for 4 weeks.

4.3 Enlarged adenoids and tonsillitis

In childhood, chronic obstruction of the airways in the back of the nose is generally due to too much lymphatic tissue at the back of the pharynx, called enlarged adenoids. Although both lymphatic growths and enlarged tonsils tend to shrink by themselves, they often prevent children from achieving the stabilised state of health and resistance to infection that most youngsters develop by age 5. A constantly open mouth and poor air circulation in the affected area are invitations to illness.

Symptoms

- Open mouth, hanging lower jaw, characteristically sleepy expression
- Impaired breathing through the nose
- Snoring (even interrupted breathing), resulting in sleep deprivation

Complications

- Inflammation of the middle ear (otitis media) (see page 33)
- Impaired hearing that may also delay the development of speech
- Paranasal sinusitis
- Bronchitis

How you can help

- 2–3 salt-water baths a week.
- For older children, 2 sessions of steam inhalation a day or nasal rinsing (see page 65).
- Drinking 3 cups of horsetail (equisetum) tea a day.
- Mustard poultices can be applied to the soles of the feet (see page 309) once daily in the evening, but be careful with children with sensitive skin.
- Ginger-salt footbaths (see page 308).
- Try to increase your child's respiratory capacity with gradually increasing pressure. First, have them blow repeatedly into a lightweight paper whistle. Later, move on to toy balloons or an Otovent nasal balloon.
- It can sometimes help to avoid milk completely to reduce protein intake. Bananas, too, can cause mucous obstructions. However, if you are reducing a toddler's milk intake, it's important to ensure they have adequate calcium and protein: yoghurt or cheese cause less

mucous obstruction than milk.
- Have your child sing and hum a lot.
- A vacation by the sea can often help.
- **If you are concerned about your child or see no improvement after 4–6 weeks of home treatments, it is time to consult a doctor.**

Remedies
- Citrus e fructibus/Cydonia e fructibus 10% solution. Add 7 drops of this solution to 5 ml physiological saline solution (0.9% NaCl). Use the dilution as a nasal spray 4–5 times a day for at least 6 weeks.
- Calcium Quercus glob. velati, 5–10 globules 3 times a day, when allergies are also present.
- Berberis/Quartz glob. velati, 5–10 globules 3 times a day for copious, very liquid nasal discharge.
- Archangelica comp. glob. velati, 5–10 globules 3 times a day to strengthen the adenoids.
- Barium comp. 1 pea-sized portion 3 times a day, for fluid accumulation in the middle ear.

Surgical removal
In severe cases, surgical removal of the adenoids may be unavoidable. This operation is always recommended if the symptoms are impacting on your child's physical and emotional well-being, particularly where there are signs of deafness or speech not developing normally. This operation is usually performed on an outpatient basis. Routine surgical insertion of ear tubes through the eardrum into the middle ear is not always advisable; discuss the options with your doctor on an individual basis.

Polyps sometimes grow back, especially if surgery is performed before your child's third birthday. After the operation, it is important to hum a lot with your child to encourage them to keep their mouth closed and breathe through their nose.

The *palatine tonsils* are important organs in the body's defence against infection and should be removed only in truly urgent cases; a few bouts of tonsillitis do not warrant this procedure and are no cause for alarm.

4.4 Coughs, croup and bronchitis

Coughing is a protective reaction to accumulation of mucus, irritation due to inflammation in the trachea or bronchi or more rarely an inhaled foreign object (see page 15).

A cough that lasts longer than 2 weeks should be watched carefully. Take your child's temperature each morning and evening for a week and then consult your doctor if the cough persists.

Cough symptoms
Long bouts of coughing
Coughs that last approximately half a minute and occur more than half an hour apart suggest whooping cough (see page 145).

Cough after exposure to measles
Coughing, nasal discharge and a slight temperature 10–14 days after exposure to measles suggest that your child is also coming down with the measles. Avoid exposing children under 1 year old and only expose other children who might contract the disease if their parents give explicit consent. Call ahead before taking a child with measles to your doctor's surgery.

Continuous coughing at night
Coughing that continues for hours (often only at night) with no other signs of discomfort is often simply due to minor irritation of the airways. Treat it by humidifying the air in your child's room (see page 64) and as for viral infections

(see page 66). Children are often much less bothered by their own coughing than the adults whose sleep they disturb.

Sudden bout of coughing
A sudden bout of coughing, especially if it occurs during the day, with no warning signs and accompanied by gagging, respiratory distress, rasping sounds during inhalation and exhalation, and spasmodic 'whistling', especially while exhaling, suggest that your child has inhaled a foreign object (see page 15).
Always call the nearest hospital Accident and Emergency department if you suspect that your child has inhaled a foreign object into their lungs.

Barking cough
A cough that sounds like a dog's bark, accompanied by respiratory distress and a harsh, rasping sound during inhalation, is due to swelling around the vocal cords and suggests croup (see page 72).

Inhalation with stridor and respiratory distress
Inhalation with stridor (a high-pitched wheezing sound caused by disrupted airflow) together with intercostal retraction (inward movement of the muscles between the ribs) and retraction at the neck

above the breastbone, can suggest the following:

- *Choking:* bits of food may be causing reflexive closing of the vocal chords. Calm your child and clap their back between the shoulder blades.
- *Croup:* (see page 72).
- *Calcium deficiency (rickets):* occasionally rickets results in these symptoms in children between the ages of 3 and 18 months. (See Section 13.11, page 255.) **Consult your doctor immediately.**

Muffled sound and obstructed air entry when breathing

A child who feels terrible, has increasing difficulty in breathing and speaking, often accompanied by sore throat, increased salivation, an inability to swallow, and has blue lips and nails and a high fever, is showing signs of **epiglottitis**. Another early sign of epiglottitis can be sudden refusal of food due to pain.

Due to the danger of suffocation, this is a medical emergency. Call emergency services or take your child to your nearest hospital Accident and Emergency department immediately.

On the way to the hospital, allow your child to sit up if it helps them breathe better.

Hoarseness or loss of voice

Inflammation and irritation of the vocal chords can be due to an infection of the air passages but may also result from overuse of the voice.

Chronic hoarseness may be caused by nodules on the vocal cords and is diagnosed by an ENT (ear, nose and throat) specialist.

Snoring sound while inhaling

This sound occurs when your child's tongue is relaxed and resting on the lower pharynx. It disappears when your child is turned on their side.

Hawking, rasping or rattling sounds while inhaling

Unless accompanied by high fever and flaring nostrils, these sounds are harmless and indicate simply that mucus has accumulated somewhere in the pharynx.

Subtle singing or 'whistling' sound while exhaling

When exhalation takes longer than inhalation, this sound is a sign of obstructive or asthmatic bronchitis (see page 73).

Flaring nostrils

Flaring nostrils (the sides of the lower part of the nose that move out as your child inhales and vice versa) indicate that your child is not getting enough air, either because the airways are partially blocked or because portions of the lungs are not functioning due to illness. When accompanied by heavy breathing, high fever, coughing and dark lips but no unusual respiratory sounds, flaring nostrils are often a sign of pneumonia (see page 78).

Reduced breathing movement of the ribcage and breathing difficulty

When accompanied by high fever and flaring nostrils, these symptoms suggest pneumonia (or pleurisy, especially if exhalation is jerky). An inhaled foreign object can also cause decreased breathing motions on one side. **Regardless of the cause, this symptom requires treatment by a doctor.**

Croup (acute laryngitis)

Croup may be preceded by flu or other infection, a walk in an easterly wind, excitement or a change in weather. Croup cases increase markedly in late autumn (November). Children just learning to talk are most frequently affected, which makes sense in view of the heavy demands placed on their speech organs.

Symptoms

- A loud barking cough and rasping inhalation (stridor) are sure signs of an inflammatory swelling of the mucous membranes around the vocal cords.
- The characteristic croup cough typically begins when the child is asleep (generally between 11:00 pm and 1:00 am). It is less likely to start during the day.
- Children are often frightened because of their difficulty in breathing.

Stages of croup

- *Stage 1:* Barking cough.
- *Stage 2:* Stridor (see above) is slight when the child is at rest, more severe with movement or excitement.
- *Stage 3:* More severe stridor at rest, flaring nostrils, retractions of the suprasternal notch (the base of neck above the breastbone) and between the ribs, tension in the auxiliary breathing muscles in neck and shoulder.
- *Stage 4:* Symptoms from the previous stages increase. The child is very restless and has blue lips and fingernails, and their pulse rate increases to 150 per minute or higher. They may lose consciousness. They appear more calm, despite difficulty with breathing.

When to seek medical advice

If this is your first experience of croup, you should take your child to your doctor or the nearest hospital Accident and Emergency department immediately, where you will learn to recognise the different degrees of severity of the illness in case the croup recurs.

Experienced parents can deal with Stages 1 and 2 at home. **Consult your doctor, however if your child has a high fever.**

If Stage 3 lasts more than 10 minutes or turns into Stage 4, always take your child straight to the nearest hospital Accident and Emergency department, where more intensive measures often produce improvement and an intubation can be performed if your child's condition continues to worsen. In this procedure, performed under anesthesia, a plastic tube is inserted through the nose or mouth into the trachea to prevent further narrowing. **If the epiglottis is inflamed (see page 71), the risk of suffocation is high and this procedure must always performed immediately.**

Due to the alarming nature of croup, we would not recommend consulting with your doctor by telephone. It is also essential to rule out the possibility of rachitic tetany (see page 257).

How you can help

- Pick up your child and comfort them: feeling their throat swelling closed is frightening for children.
- Wrap your child in a blanket and stand with them by an open window or out on a balcony so they can breathe the cold night air. In most cases, this will help your child breathe more easily and they will calm down.
- If two adults are available, one should fetch a vaporiser or, alternatively, a couple of damp cloths to hang around your child's bed, as well as a pot of hot water to put close by in a safe place on the floor.
- Turning on the hot shower in the bathroom is a quick way to produce hot, moist air for your child to inhale.
- Bryonia Spongia comp. dilution. Add 10 drops to warm herbal tea with honey.

Bronchitis

If your child coughs a lot or has frequent bouts of bronchitis, you may wonder if they have asthma. However, note that there are differences between the two. Bronchitis often follows one of the upper respiratory infections described previously and may be prevented by careful treatment of the primary infection (see page 74).

Symptoms

- Preceded by a simple cold
- Persistent upper respiratory symptoms (see page 69)
- Possible recurrence of fever
- Cough that is deep-seated, long-lasting and increasingly noisy and laboured
- Abnormal breathing sounds and coughing
- Respiratory obstruction

How you can help

- Have your child inhale physiological saline solution (0.9% NaCl) from a damp cloth or try steam inhalation (see page 312).
- Apply a powdered ginger or honey compress to your child's chest in the middle of the day (see page 300).
- At night, apply a chest compress using 5–10% lavender oil or thyme oil.
- Give any child over age 1 plenty of warm thyme or sage tea with honey.

Remedies

- Tartarus stibiatus comp. 1 pea-sized portion 3–6 times a day for very tough mucus.
- Bryonia 4X, 5 drops 3–6 times a day, in a little tea, for abundant loose mucus.
- Bronchi Plantago glob. velati, 5 globules 3–6 times a day for obstructive (spastic) bronchitis.

Obstructive bronchitis

This usually affects infants and is rarer in toddlers. It is typically a viral infection in which swelling of the mucous membranes displaces the bronchi and obstructs respiration. At the same age, a harmless cough, teething or change in weather can show similar symptoms without lasting effects. Usually the bronchitis disappears after a year or two.

Obstructive bronchitis is not necessarily a precursor of asthma but does not preclude it. Children with early childhood asthma may have a temporary tendency towards obstructive bronchitis, but are more likely to have allergies in either their individual medical history (atopic dermatitis) or their family history (hay fever, bronchial asthma).

'Bronchial hyperresponsiveness' is a term increasingly used when children develop obstructive bronchitis on the heels of every cold, but a diagnosis of asthma would still be premature.

Symptoms

- The child exhales slowly and with difficulty, and their chest and nostrils flare (see page 79).
- If you listen close to their nose, you can hear a combination of quiet 'whistling' and gentle bubbling sounds (reminiscent of the

sound of simmering water or the wheezy asthmatic breathing of older people) as they exhale.

- Dry cough or coughing phlegm, sometimes even vomiting.
- Some children are cheerful, although exerting themselves; others appear to be very ill.
- A fever is more common with simple bronchitis.
- Severe respiratory distress is a sign that the smallest bronchi are involved (bronchiolitis).

How you can help

- The first time you experience these symptoms in your child, consult your doctor, who will help you learn to evaluate your child's condition. Severe cases of obstructive bronchitis always need urgent treatment or even hospitalisation.
- Fresh air is important during the treatment, and you can even apply the poultice outside the house if you wrap your child up warmly and watch them carefully.
- Keep your child's surroundings calm, warm and relaxed.
- Warm compress around the chest with 5–10% lavender and eucalyptus oils (see page 301).
- The most effective home remedy is a chest poultice made with ground ginger or mustard. If you have experienced

its soothing effects, you will know that it is worth the effort to make it. **It is a very strong treatment and should be used only if you have mastered the technique and only on the advice of your child's doctor. Never apply one of these poultices to a child who is less than 4 months old, has overly sensitive skin or is allergy-prone.** Ginger or mustard poultices work by increasing perfusion in the skin over the ribcage, which stimulates breathing, makes secretions more fluid (allowing them to be coughed up more easily) and, in older children, relaxes cramped bronchial muscles. Ginger is somewhat milder and more warming than mustard. (For instructions on how to make these poultices, see page 293).

Remedies

- As for bronchitis (see page 74)
- Inhalations of:
- Saline solution 0.9% NaCl and Tabacum Cupro cultum Rh 3X Dilution 1 ml, 3–6 times daily for mild cases.
- Saline solution 0.9% NaCl 2 ml, with the addition of Salbutamol if prescribed by your child's doctor and if the above-listed measures and inhalations have not resulted in any improvement.

- Cuprum aceticum 4X, 5 globules 3–6 times a day (this treatment may be continued during convalescence and stabilisation).
- Nicotiana comp. glob. velati, 3–5 globules as frequently as every half hour, for a dry, spastic cough.
- Bryonia comp. glob. velati, 5 globules 3–6 times per day, for a fever with abundant mucus production.

4.5 Asthma

Although the symptoms of asthma are quite similar to those of obstructive bronchitis, asthma can be triggered more easily. Toddlers might breathe with difficulty for no apparent reason, and school children might cough every night during sleep, waking up tired and exhausted. They are ill more often than 'average' children and might not like to take part in PE lessons. They tire quickly, especially in winter.

These children may have asthma (i.e. an inflammatory allergic swelling in the bronchi that will persist during 'healthy' periods). The swelling can be confirmed clinically in children from age 6 with a spirometry test. Younger children are diagnosed by the symptoms.

The attacks are triggered by a variety of causes, such as dust mite excrement in house dust, pollen, the spores of fungi or animal dander. The attacks can worsen in cold air, fog, dust or tobacco smoke, or after physical exertion, and sometimes because of emotional issues. Children with asthma often avoid exertion, which some parents misinterpret as laziness.

There are reports of an increase of symptoms in the early morning. At the beginning of an attack, some patients often have a sensation of heaviness in the chest. This is quickly followed by breathing problems. Occasionally, asthma disappears spontaneously during adolescence. (See also Section 6.15.)

Drug therapy, whether short- or long-term, must be prescribed by your doctor, who will decide whether to use the allopathic medications typically prescribed in paediatric asthma (bronchodilators, cortisone and others) and/or homeopathic or anthroposophic medications. Over-medication is not uncommon in asthma cases and may cause hormonal side effects or chronic circulatory problems. In some cases, parents or children downplay the severity of the asthmatic symptoms out of concern over possible side effects. However, it is vital to make your child's well-being the highest priority and you should always seek medical advice before making decisions about medication.

In recent years, asthma education has begun to play a major role in treatment. Asthmatic children and their parents can learn to assess the severity of symptoms and the appropriate treatment. The goal is to minimise the impact of the illness and allow the patient to enjoy a normally active life.

Whether in individual conversations with your child's doctor or in a group session, learning to deal with anxiety is one of the most important elements in asthma education and is especially applicable to your child's immediate surroundings. Either emotional upheaval or a cold can trigger an asthma attack, and calming a young child can significantly reduce its severity. Older children can learn and use breathing and relaxation exercises. The inner 'victory' of children accepting and learning to deal with their condition is a significant step towards lessening their symptoms.

Sports in groups directed by specialists, as well as movement therapy like curative eurythmy (see page 242), can help to strengthen breathing and give emotional support.

Symptoms
- Dry, nagging, nervous cough
- Retractions between the ribs
- Laboured breathing, even severe breathlessness
- During an attack, leaning forwards with support helps breathing
- Restlessness and fear
- Possibly tiring quickly

How you can help
- For acute symptoms, follow the measures described under *Obstructive bronchitis* (page 75).

Remedies
- In our experience, the following often reduce the need for medication:
- Ground mustard or grated ginger poultices, especially for attacks triggered by infections (see page 298).
- For asthma attacks due to other causes, try lavender oil wraps (made, if needed, with hot, moist compresses) or hot horsetail (equisetum) wraps (see page 311).
- During an attack, give plenty of warm fluids, such as herb tea. Fizzy drinks are unhelpful, as your child will usually gulp air into the stomach while drinking them. Cold drinks can act as a trigger.
- Skilful use of rhythmical massage as indicated by Ita Wegman,

77

such as respiratory rubs and torso and calf massages, can be very helpful during asthma attacks.[1] To give a respiratory rub, stand behind your child, who should bend slightly forwards and support or rest their head and arms on a table in front of them. Timing the strokes to your child's breathing, lift your hands and arms when they inhale and brush lightly downwards with your hands on either side of their spine as they exhale.

• Rest, warmth and relaxation are helpful.

• Many children are helped by a prescribed course of copper ointment compresses applied to the area of the body above the kidneys every evening (Cuprum metallicum praep. 0.1% ointment or red copper ointment).

• Astringent oak bark or sage tea in the morning is a long-term constitutional aid to take on waking up.

• Bitter veronica tea in the evening helps with falling asleep and is another long-term constitutional aid.

4.6 Pneumonia

Pneumonia often develops from a prior cold or bronchitis, but can appear without earlier illness. If your child is diagnosed with pneumonia it can be very frightening, but in kindergarten-age children, or even some older children, in most cases the course of the illness is not especially dangerous. Greater caution is advised in the case of infants or in older children weakened by other acute or chronic illnesses.

Pneumonia must be diagnosed and treated by your family doctor or paediatrician. For children at risk or when the quality of care cannot be guaranteed at home, your doctor will recommend hospitalisation. A doctor experienced in complementary medicine may be able to avoid using antibiotics. For many years, we have not prescribed antibiotics for either hospitalised patients or outpatients except in high-risk or unusually severe cases, or on the family's request.

In our experience, one of the advantages of antibiotic-free treatment is that the pneumonia very rarely recurs. The purpose of such treatment is to help the body learn to respond more flexibly to environmental influences and to achieve a new level of stability by coming to grips with the illness. Immediately administering antibiotics blocks the normal course of the disease and denies the organism an opportunity to exercise its own forces of resistance and strengthen them to fight future infections.

If we view illness only as something to be eliminated as quickly as possible, of course we will prefer antibiotic treatment, but if we acknowledge it as an opportunity for the body to learn (i.e. as a process that the body itself seeks out in order to apply its own forces and exercise its defences) we will attempt to support and soothe the patient without immediately opting for suppressive therapies. This supportive approach respects the quality of the patient's future health and the individuality of the child whose forces and assets work together with the treatment we provide.

Symptoms
- Usually typical symptoms of a cold
- Prolonged or rising fever
- Generally feeling worse
- Coughing, initially hacking, later with phlegm
- Shortness of breath, possibly

leaning forward with support to help breathing
- Flaring nostrils (the sides of the lower part of the nose move out as your child inhales and vice versa)
- Dark-red lips, in severe cases turning blue

How you can help
- **If you suspect pneumonia, always seek medical advice.** If your doctor considers your child well enough to be treated at home, the following can be helpful.
- Follow the same measures described in Section 4.2 on viral infections (see page 66), adapted as needed to the child's weakened condition.
- When coughing is the dominant symptom, especially in children who are quite thin, rubbing the chest with 10% lavender or thyme oil (see page 302) or with ointments containing etheric oils of camphor, eucalyptus or the like, can be effective.
- For significant fluid accumulation in the bronchi or on the lungs, apply warm, damp compresses made with horsetail (equisetum) tea or thick quark (fermented skimmed milk; see page 303).
- For respiratory spasms, use chest

poultices made with ground mustard or ginger (see pages 298 and 300). Use only after consulting your doctor.

• After the acute symptoms disappear, a recuperation time of up to 4 weeks is often needed.

Remedies

• Pneumodoron 1 and 2, initially alternating 5 drops hourly. In the evenings do not give Pneumodoron 2, to avoid sleep disturbance.
• Pulsatilla 12X, 5 globules 3–6 times a day if emotionally upset.
• Apis/Belladonna glob. velati, 5 globules 3–6 times a day, only with high fever.
• Rose iron/Graphit, glob. velati, 5–10 globules 3 times a day for about 4 weeks to help convalescence.

4.7 Hay fever

Hay fever is an allergic reaction stimulated by a high pollen count and is at its worst during the summer, especially when it is warm and windy. Common triggers are grasses, trees or flowers, dust mite excrement in house dust, and certain fungi. Hay fever, especially if accompanied by asthmatic symptoms, is often a tremendous burden, and people are always in search of treatments with lasting effects.

Symptoms

• Runny nose
• Swollen, red and possibly itching nasal mucous membranes
• Impaired breathing through the nose
• Red and itchy mucous membranes inside the eyelids

How you can help

• If possible, regularly spend time by the seaside: allergen-poor sea air is beneficial and has strengthening effects.
• Eating a daily spoonful of local honey (preferably raw, from natural beeswax honeycomb), which has been produced using pollen from local flowers, can be effective. This treatment must be continued throughout the year.
• Rinsing the nasal passages twice a day (see page 65).

Remedies

• From age 10, regular inhalation treatments with an extract of lemon and quince (commercially available as Gencydo 0.1% and Citrus e. fruct./ Cydonia e. fruct. 2X/2X). This treatment should begin in early spring, to prevent symptoms before they start.

- From age 6, topical applications of Gencydo 0.1% drops (in both the nose and the eyes) are also effective.
- Echinacea/Quartz comp. eye-drops, applied locally several times a day, relieve irritation and fight inflammation in the early stages of infection.
- Weleda Hay Fever spray, 2 to 3 times a day.
- Many patients benefit from additional constitutional treat-ment (see page 248) over a few years, which may be prescribed by your doctor.

Desensitisation

A treatment we recommend on a few occasions is desensitisation. This consists of a series of injec-tions of specially produced allergen extracts. After testing to identify the patient's allergies, gradually increasing doses of the allergen are injected into the surface of the skin. This approach is very effec-tive for those allergic only to single, specific plants but less effective for people who have multiple allergies or are allergic to house dust, which is almost impossible to avoid. One disadvantage of this treatment, which must be continued for at least 3 years, is the need for frequent injections.

There is also always the chance that an injection may provoke a severe allergic reaction. Many people also find that they become sensitive to other allergens either during or after successful desensitisation to the original allergen; that is, their symptoms return because they have become allergic to something else.

It is interesting to note that studies have shown that an 'anthroposophical lifestyle' that includes not only Waldorf education but also biodynamic food, plenty of outdoor play in rural or natural surroundings and cultivating a healthy sleep/wake rhythm contributes to preventing allergies.[2]

4.8 Young children's susceptibility to infection

Parents of children who have just entered kindergarten often lament that their children spend no more than a couple of days at school before they're sick and stuck at home again. If it is any consolation, you can expect this pattern to persist for one or at most two winters, after which your child's immune system will grow stronger and learn to handle these frequent infections and ward them off. In other words, their body goes through a learning process that leads to a more stable state of health. That is why it is important to let children have sufficient time to properly recuperate after an acute infection.

In this 'forest' of minor infections, the familiar childhood diseases stick out like a few towering trees. In some instances, they seem to put an end to a long string of infections.

If there are younger siblings at home, they may be infected too, which gives parents cause for concern because babies' immune systems are still undeveloped. In fact, however, as anyone who has three or more children can confirm, the youngest ones who go through the classic childhood illnesses at an early age are usually healthiest later on, because they have had to struggle so intensely with these infections.

But we must not assume that immature immune systems and the possibility of contagion are the only factors in the development of infections. Children's illnesses often begin the day after a fall down the stairs, a birthday party, a long car trip or going to a movie. In the first instance, parents are understandably concerned that a fall and the illness may be related, and of course a doctor needs to rule out unex-pected consequences of a head injury. In most cases, however, the illness is simply the young body's response to being overwhelmed by some unaccustomed event, and 'catching' an illness restores the balance.

Normally, a young child is intensely involved with their immediate surroundings and identifies strongly with it. As a result, any unexpected event tends to throw the child back in on themselves in a way that is actively painful. Through such incidents, the soul's experience of itself in the body is both taxed and constrained, producing an emotional 'chill' that the child's immature constitution is not ready to deal with. In these situations, both physical and emotional warmth are healing.

Anything we can do to help the child feel comfortable in their body supports their sympathetic relationship with their surroundings, and love and attention warm and strengthen the body. From this perspective, we can approach the treatment of infections differently, soothing the child's way through illness rather than suppressing symptoms with medication. We see the illness and the triggering event as an opportunity to strengthen and harmonise the child's constitution.

4.9 Breathing as an expression of psychological activity

Even in infants and toddlers, we can observe that respiration clearly shifts from expansive exhalation and relaxation during sleep to deep inhalation in the waking state. The various states we observe in children's daily lives – the contraction of pain and the expansive release of joy, hopeful sighs of relief, limp resignation, nimble activity and sudden cessation of movement – are all accompanied by their own respiratory rhythms that adapt dynamically to the subtlest stirrings of the child's soul. Nothing is more informative about another person's momentary emotional state than their breathing.

In the waking state, the soul is drawn in or 'inhaled' into the body, ready to sense and move, to experience and act, to love and hate. In sleep, the soul leaves behind a peacefully resting 'remnant': the body lies tired and heavy in bed, and the gentle ebb and flow of the breath belongs completely to the body's life processes. The soul no longer supports conscious activity and conveys no expressions of emotion.

If we consider the possibilities for abnormal changes in respiration as described in previous sections, we note that disturbances in the ability to move air hinder the soul's free interaction with its environment. This phenomenon is most evident in asthma (see page 76).

But other disturbances also influence breathing, for example, slight changes in the acidity of the blood, usually related to heart, lung or kidney diseases. Damage to the nervous system may also change the character of respiration, as do certain drugs, such as barbiturates, which depress respiration.

Just as we speak of a warmth-body in connection with the activity of the human 'I', we can also see the air-body (regulated by respiration) as directly related to the life of the human soul. On the one hand, this air-body is connected to the entire metabolism through gaseous exchange and assorted buffer systems in the blood. On the other hand, it enables the activity of a human soul to express itself in a body. After all, the very nature of emotional experience is rhythmical alternation between attempts to be self-contained and becoming receptive to the concerns of one's surroundings.

The laws of soul activity (sympathy and antipathy, the dynamics of pleasure and pain, laughing and crying) correspond to the inherent laws and dynamics of air: pressure and suction, concentration and dilution, the ability to expand in all directions yet become concentrated again under appropriate conditions of pressure. Thus healthy breathing supports the soul's ability to express itself freely. Conversely, quiet conversations, positive emotional input or restful, comforting experiences can help restore order to disturbed respiration.

The alternation between waking and sleeping is repeated in miniature in each breath we take. Sleeping corresponds to the outpouring of exhalation, while waking (which isolates a certain amount of air from the environment, as it were) corresponds to inhalation. The great transformations of birth and death are also linked to breathing. With a baby's first breath, the soul activity that supports consciousness pervades the child's body, which moments before was still heavy, dark, newly born. At the same instant, the baby's skin turns pink, their eyes open and they utter their first cry. And in a dying person's last unutterably long and gentle exhalation, we experience their final exit from a body that has become unusable.

5. Vomiting, Diarrhoea and Constipation

The digestive system of infants and toddlers develops over the course of their first few years and only gradually achieves full functionality. For example, the intestinal flora unique to each individual develops during the first three years of life. This is an important accomplishment in physiological development, because healthy digestion means that ingested food is completely transformed into endogenous substance. When short-term digestive problems develop, it is important to pay attention to them to avoid development of long-term disorders. Emotionally stressful, 'undigested' experiences can also lead to digestive symptoms.

When assessing digestive disturbances at home, vomiting, diarrhoea and constipation are the most important symptoms to consider. For clarity, we will begin by defining these terms:

- **Vomiting:** At least one quarter of your child's last meal comes up again. If only 1 or 2 mouthfuls are regurgitated it is referred to as possetting or 'spitting up'.
- **Diarrhoea:** Here, not only the frequency (for example, 6–10 times a day), but also the quantity (a few squirts or a cupful), colour (yellow, grey, green, brown, black, bloody etc.) and consistency (watery, runny, loose, mushy) are important. 2 soft stools in 1 day, for example, do not constitute diarrhoea. Breast-fed babies can poo between once in 10 days to 10 times a day.

Vomiting and diarrhoea are often important attempts at self-healing, protecting the body from harmful influences. But because they entail losses of fluids and salts, the cause of the disturbance must be recognised and treated promptly.

- **Constipation:** Constipation is present when bowel-movement frequency is reduced to less than once every 3 days, emptying the bowels takes considerable effort, and faeces are hard and possibly lumpy. It is a very troublesome condition. In chronic cases, it is also affected by your child's emotional state. Constipation that requires treatment is very uncommon in babies who are being breast-fed (see page 190).

5.1 Vomiting and diarrhoea

Occasional vomiting in infants

Causes
- Eating too much or too quickly
- Too much air in the stomach
- Excitement
- Food that has gone slightly bad
- A cold, irritation of the throat or palate, teething etc.
- During teething, your baby may simply tolerate less food than usual. This is not worrisome; it will not result in long-term failure to thrive.

How you can help
- Anti-flatulence measures (see page 41).
- When your baby has an upper respiratory infection, administering salt nasal drops (0.9% NaCl) before nursing may help.
- When your baby's oral mucous membranes are irritated, your paediatrician may prescribe diluted mouth balsam (Wala Mundbalsam gel) to brush on the inside of their mouth 15 minutes before feeding.

Simple gastrointestinal infections, diarrhoea

Simple gastrointestinal infections and diarrhoea have many causes, such as ingesting milk that has been standing around too long, foods that are slightly 'off', viruses and bacteria.

Although either viruses (e.g. rotavirus, norovirus, adenovirus) or bacteria (e.g. salmonella or specific strains of E. coli) may be the cause of diarrhoea, stool tests to determine which pathogen is involved are necessary only in exceptional cases or if complications occur. The body expels these 'foreign irritants' by vomiting.

Symptoms
- Vomiting, usually to begin with
- Sometimes the child is pale and not well some hours beforehand
- Sometimes diarrhoea begins after 1 or 2 days

- A light to high fever
- Stomachache

Warning signs requiring an immediate visit to the doctor or hospital

- Your overall impression of your child is important. Does your child seem merely irritated by their symptoms or are they totally different from usual?
- Are they noticeably quiet, weak or showing apathy?
- Signs of dehydration: rings around their eyes, dry tongue, hard abdomen when touched, infrequent urination, sunken fontanelle of infants.
- High fever around 40°C/104°F
- Blood mixed with the stools
- Blood in urine after diarrhoea
- Depending on the circumstances, the doctor will decide whether further treatment at home is possible or whether your child needs an intravenous infusion.

How you can help

- It is vital to replace lost fluids and salts during gastrointestinal infections and diarrhoea. The following measures will help:
- Continue feeding breastfed infants as usual. For formula-fed infants, if your doctor recommends it, dilute the feed to about half the concentration.
- Additionally, offer herb tea. For young infants fennel tea is best; from 6 months onwards infants can also have very dilute chamomile, rosehip, blackberry-leaf tea or tea made with dried apples. Some children prefer cold tea or still water instead. Only add juice or milk in tiny quantities to make it look more appetising to your child if they are reluctant to drink it.
- A commercial rehydration mixture from your pharmacy has the best possible ingredients for replacing lost salt and minerals. However, they taste sweet-salty and many children do not like them.
- If the tea has been tolerated, after some hours, offer infants who are already esrablished on solid food thin cream of rice. Add 3–4 g rice powder to 100 ml water (1 tsp to half a US cup).
- Toddlers and school-age children can be offered rusks, breadsticks, lightly salted rice or oat porridge.
- If the vomiting has stopped, offer older infants, toddlers and school-age children puréed carrots, grated apple, mashed banana, white bread or rolls, toast or crackers, or mashed potatoes (without milk), pasta without eggs or blueberry juice.

- The carrots, although they should make the stools somewhat more solid, typically look the same 'coming out as going in'. Without carrots, the stools generally remain loose, stringy and without much volume.
- When the diarrhoea has improved, continue with a low-fat diet: natural yoghurt, quark, diluted milk, thinly spread butter. Yoghurt is especially good because the lactobacilli in it support normalisation of the intestinal flora.

Remedies

- *For vomiting and nausea:* Nux vomicae semine 6X or 12X glob. velati, initially 5 globules as frequently as every half hour.
- *For infants:* Geum urbanum Rh 3X, 5 drops given approximately as often as diarrhoea occurs.
- *For older children:* Bolus alba comp. Powder, ½–1 teaspoon dissolved in half a cup of tea, taken in sips 1–2 times a day.
- *For children who are pale and cool and have abdominal cramps:* Veratrum album radice 6X glob. velati, 5 globules 3–6 times a day.
- *For abdominal cramping:* Nicotiana comp. glob. velati, 5 globules as frequently as every half hour.
- *For older children, as an extra measure if still required:* Carbo betulae comp. capsules, dispersed in herbal tea.

Acetonemic (ketonic) vomiting

For unknown reasons, some children between the ages of 2 and 10 are susceptible to disruptions in fat breakdown, which cause the production of acetone and similar compounds. If your child is vomiting for this reason and you have an acute sense of smell, you might notice an apple-like odour as soon as you enter your child's room.

If this is your child's first bout of acetonemic vomiting, consult your doctor. In future you will be able to assess the situation yourself. It's essential to provide sugar and fluids to restore metabolic balance. However, your child may need an intravenous infusion in hospital if there are signs of dehydration (see page 87).

Symptoms

- Convulsive vomiting up to 50 times a day
- Abdominal wall is soft but not tender to the touch
- Severe abdominal pain may be present several hours before vomiting begins
- Relatively few bowel movements

How you can help

- Every 10 minutes, give your child a sip of herb tea with 5% glucose or sugar added (i.e. 1 teaspoon per 100 ml / half a cup). Fennel or chamomile teas are suitable; acidic teas such as mallow or peppermint are not as good. The sugar in the tea restores the metabolic balance. Don't worry if your child vomits several more times after drinking the tea. Reassure them, tell them they'll feel better soon and urge them to take the next sip of tea slowly. They'll keep down at least some of it. After an hour or 2, slowly increase the amounts you give your child to drink until they can keep down a cup of sweetened tea at a time.

- Instead of straight sweetened tea, you may give your child either still mineral water with glucose or a commercial rehydration mixture from your pharmacy, which has the advantage of replacing lost salt and minerals.

- Although children who have been vomiting are often given Coca-Cola and salted crisps, we do not recommend this practice. Coke, which contains phosphates and caffeine, is a stimulant and therefore not a suitable drink for children, especially those prone to acetonemic vomiting, because their vegetative functions are less stable than normal.

- Once the vomiting has stopped, you can give your child some dry rusks in addition to the tea. Over the following days, their diet should be bland and fat-free.

- Apply a warm chamomile or oxalis compress (see page 305) to your child's abdomen.

- **If the vomiting persists for more than a few hours in spite of these measures, it is advisable to consult your doctor. You should certainly do so if your child develops a dry tongue and rings around their eyes, as there may be a need for an immediate intravenous infusion.**

Remedies

- Nux vomica e semine 6X or 12X glob. velati, 5 globules half-hourly in acute cases.

- As a constitutional remedy, Wala Gentiana Stomach pellets, glob. velati or Chelidonium/Colocynthis glob. velati, 5–10 globules 3 times a day before meals, for at least 1 month.

Other causes of vomiting

- If your child vomits **after a fall or head injury,** call the emergency services or take them to your nearest hospital Accident and Emergency department.

- For vomiting **after a sudden fright or upset,** calm your child and keep them warm. If the shock seems serious, have them examined by a doctor.
- **If occasional vomiting occurs at increasingly frequent intervals and is accompanied by headache**, ask your doctor to perform a neurological examination.

5.2 Chronic constipation

When your child is constipated, their entire large intestine is packed full and must be emptied. Constipation may be caused by foods such as white bread, chocolate, white rice, carrots or too few unsaturated fats like oils or margarine. Having too little to drink is also a culprit. Changes to habits or rhythms, for example travel, can cause constipation. Sometimes, painful anal fissures cause constipation – these can even occur in toddlers. A visit to the doctor is definitely in order if your child repeatedly retains their stools for longer than usual, with or without soiling their underwear. Behavioural and emotional reasons must also be explored.

Symptoms
- Reduced frequency of stools (i.e. fewer than 1 every 3 days)

- The above together with difficult bowel movements and balls of hardened faeces
- Flatulence and bulging stomach
- Anal fissures (possibly)
- Feeling unhappy (possibly)

How you can help
- Suppositories can be used, but their stool-softening effects are often inadequate.
- It is important to empty the entire large intestine, not just the rectum. Feel the abdomen to check how well the enema has worked. **Repeated use of enemas and suppositories can lead to dependency, so it is a good idea to talk to your doctor about how often they should be used.**
- The next step is to make a few sensible dietary changes:
- It is important to drink plenty.
- Sometimes it is enough to replace a couple of servings of milk with peppermint tea in the mornings.
- Ensure your child has adequate fibre in their diet. e.g. fruit, vegetables, muesli and wholemeal produce.
- If your child becomes constipated on oat cereals and wholegrain bread, try reducing the amount of fibre in their diet, especially if wind and stomachaches are frequent problems.

- Many children need more fat in their diet.
- Avoid *'binding' foods,* e.g. cocoa, bananas, white bread or rolls, black tea, blueberries, margarine and possibly milk.
- *Laxative foods* include rhubarb, stewed prunes, figs, buttermilk, yoghurt, sour milk, mineral water, orange juice, milk sugar (lactose), olive oil and flaxseed.
- Try a teaspoon of ground flax-seed twice a day before meals, mixed with yoghurt, soup or a little honey and 3 drops of lemon juice. Alternatively, the flaxseed can be mixed into food.
- Don't forget that the family situation can be an important factor in treating constipation. If constipation is an old, familiar problem for the older generation, a child's first missed bowel movement will have a very different impact than it will if their parents are not already sensitised to the issue.
- Regardless of family history, however, it is indisputably true that nothing is more constipating than worrying about bowel movements. In contrast, lively interest in one's surroundings has a laxative effect. If your child tends to be constipated, make sure that every day includes something exciting to look forward to, even if it is just a little surprise they prepare for someone else. This is also true of infants and toddlers, but in their case the element of anticipation and surprise must be provided through how you relate to them.
- If dietary measures fail, your doctor must determine the cause of the problem.

5.3 Learning to digest

Grace by Christian Morgenstern:
Earth who gives to us this food,
Sun who makes it ripe and good,
Dear Sun, dear Earth,
By you we live,
Our loving thanks to you we give.

The fact that a baby's gastrointestinal tract is especially susceptible to disturbances indicates that the ability to digest is acquired gradually. But what do the digestive organs have to 'learn'? What does digestion actually accomplish?

The purpose of digestion is to destroy everything that makes a food identifiable; in other words, the better the digestion, the less an ingested bit of fish or radish remains as it was. Foods can be used to build up human substance only after being broken down completely. As products of the outer world, they must 'die' in order to serve the development of human forces. If any trace of undigested protein from a different species enters the bloodstream, it triggers an acute reaction in the form of fever or allergic symptoms. The appearance of food intolerances (to gluten, milk protein or specific sugars) means that the body is no longer adequately able to transform that particular bit of the outside world into human substance.

Any dietary plan should progress from the most easily digested foods to the least digestible. Some illnesses may make it necessary to eliminate certain foods temporarily. Ideally, however, the goal should be to again learn to digest foods that once had to be avoided. The more our metabolism is able to transform all foods into human substance, the stronger and more determined we can be.

It is interesting to note that this physical work of digestion also corresponds, not coincidentally, to the ability to carry out emotional, intellectual and spiritual 'digestive' processes: we 'grit our teeth' as we tackle problems or tough assignments that initially appear 'indigestible'. It is astonishing to realise that the bodily work of digestion is actually the polar opposite of how

the human soul and spirit process the outer world.

Healthy digestion transforms mineral, plant and animal matter into human bodies, while healthy soul-spiritual digestion accomplishes just the opposite. Our attempts at recognition and understanding succeed only to the extent that we are able to submit to that which we hope to understand, *to transforming ourselves* into it, so to speak, and seeing it from the inside. In understanding and recognising something other than ourselves, *we become one with the outer world.* We must overcome our personal feelings, opinions and preferences if they are 'wrong', that is not in line with the reality that we are attempting to understand.

In digestion, the world communicates with humans on a bodily level; that is, the world is transformed into human matter and human forces, sacrificing itself so that human beings can exist. In our mental efforts, however, we communicate with the surrounding world on a soul-spiritual level, learning to understand it on its own terms, as it actually is, by overcoming ourselves and 'sacrificing' personal perspectives or erroneous opinions. These two ways of processing the outer world support each other, but they reveal the full scope of human nourishment only when seen together.

Both spiritual and physical nourishment always involve a transformation that allows development to occur. Understandably, therefore, in the Christian religion with its focus on evolution and development, the process of nourishment appears in its true and sacred significance in the Christian rite of Holy Communion.

Rudolf Steiner expressed this reality in a grace that children also enjoy saying:

The plant-seeds are quickened in
the night of the Earth,
The green herbs sprouting
through the might of the Air,
And all fruits are ripened
by the power of the Sun.
So quickens the soul in
the shrine of the Heart,
So blossoms Spirit-power
in the light of the World,
So ripens Man's strength
in the glory of God.[3]

6. Skin Diseases and Rashes

The skin reflects the entire body's state. It shows how well rested the body is, its nutritional condition and level of hydration, as well as the health of circulation, liver, kidneys, adrenals, the thyroid gland and the nervous system. Skin symptoms more or less directly reveal the activity of the living body or the person's soul and spirit. It is well known, for example, that itching can be caused by deposition of uric acid and bilirubin in the skin during metabolic disturbances of the kidneys and liver. Even more familiar are the phenomena of turning pale with fright or anxiety and blushing with shame, or the more subtle blush of pleasurable excitement. The discussion of symptoms and diseases in this chapter will help you to judge whether or not a visit to the doctor is warranted. We will also provide general guidelines for skincare and home treatment of skin diseases.

6.1 Birthmarks and pigmentation

Stork's beak marks (or salmon patches)

These are flat, superficially reddened areas of skin that appear at birth and are caused by harmless dilation of delicate blood vessels in the skin. Stork's beak marks are either located centrally/symmetrically (in the middle of the forehead, on both eyelids or eyebrows, for example) or on one side. If located centrally/symmetrically they are harmless and usually disappear in your baby's first year. One-sided marks, however, tend to remain and in a few cases can be involved with changes in other organs, making a medical examination advisable.

Strawberry marks (naevi or *haemangioma*)

Strawberry marks are soft, red, round, elevated areas of skin and can appear anywhere on the body. At birth, often only a reddened spot is conspicuous but during the first few weeks of life, the red colouration deepens and the mark rises above the general level of the skin. Deeper birthmarks can form a protruding knot, possibly with a bluish tinge. Strawberry marks generally appear (and grow larger) during the first year of life and then gradually disappear. If they are on the face, particularly near the eyes, nose or mouth, as well in bothersome locations like joints, nappy area, hands or feet, discuss treatment with your doctor.

Early treatment (cryotherapy or laser therapy) is recommended in cases where a birthmark may impact vision or increase the risk of injury. Deeper haemangiomas are uncommon but can be surgically removed. More recently, drug treatment with beta blockers has become possible, but due to its effects throughout the body, it is recommended only in exceptional cases.

Pigmented spots or hyperpigmentation

These types of spots take many forms and generally persist for a lifetime. Look for brown, bluish to black spots, possibly from birth, with or without hairs. Types include liver spots (lentigines), freckles, café-au-lait spots and Mongolian spots. Spots that are unusually asymmetrical, irregularly bounded, multi-coloured, raised or increasing in size should be checked out by a doctor or a skin specialist.

Light-coloured café-au-lait spots are usually inconspicuous, variable in size and increase up to school age. If your baby has more than 5 such spots or if they cover large areas of skin, ask your doctor about them to preclude certain rare diseases.

6.2 Jaundice (yellow skin colouration)

Jaundice in newborns

Jaundice is present to a greater or lesser extent in almost all newborn babies as long as the liver is still breaking down foetal blood pigment. Although breast-fed babies can show symptoms for some weeks, usually jaundice is harmless. However, in a small number of cases it can be the sign of an underlying health condition, so speak to your doctor if your baby is struggling to feed or you are concerned for any other reason.

Symptoms

- Varying yellow skin colouration, and the whites of the eyes are also yellow
- Difficulties with drinking milk (possibly)

How you can help

- Continue breastfeeding, if you have chosen to breastfeed.
- Speak to your doctor if you are concerned.

Remedies

- Cichorium Stanno cultum Rh 3X, 5 drops before each feed.
- In serious cases, light therapy is administered in the hospital throughout the night using special lamps together with infusions.

'Carrot juice' jaundice

Yellow skin colouration that does not also involve the whites of the eyes usually comes from eating large amounts of carrots and is totally harmless, although we would recommend consuming fewer carrots!

Cholestasis (reduction or cessation of bile flow), liver disease

For any suspected liver problems with the following symptoms, seek immediate medical help.

Symptoms

- Yellow skin colouration, including the whites of the eyes
- Greyish-white stools
- Dark shade of urine

6.3 Marbled or bluish skin

Marbling of the skin, or bluish tinged skin, are usually completely normal, especially after heavy meals, but it is important to take note of the following possible causes.

Lung or heart disease, and sepsis

If your child is displaying the following symptoms it is important to seek medical help immediately.

Symptoms

- Marbled skin
- Weak blood circulation
- Blue colouration of the lips, fingernails and feet
- Rapid breathing
- Weak or rapid pulse
- General weakness
- Raised or lowered temperature (applicable to sepsis)

Chilblains

Chilblains are the inflammation of small blood vessels in your skin in response to exposure to cold air.

Symptoms

- Blue colouration of the lips, fingernails and/or feet
- Marbling of the skin

- Painful reddish, swollen spots, especially around the joints of the fingers and toes

How you can help
- For children over the age of 1, give hot herb tea with honey.
- Dress your child in warm (woollen) clothes.
- Do not apply too much heat directly to the affected area.

6.4 Red cheeks

Children often have red cheeks as a sign of excitement, and from running around in the fresh air. This is completely normal. However, if you are concerned, red cheeks can also be a symptom of the following:
- Fever (see page 53)
- Scarlet fever (see page 133)
- Teething – usually accompanied by one-sided, painful swellings (see page 32).
- Mumps – usually accompanied by painful swellings on both sides (see page 143).

Overexposure to cold
Symptoms may emerge during a walk in the wind, for instance. Round-cheeked 6-month-olds are particularly susceptible.

Symptoms
- Reddened cheeks

- Oversensitive skin
- Tissue that feels hard to the touch

How you can help
- Rosatum Heilsalbe (best applied before exposure to cold).
- Moisturise affected skin with a fat-based cream or ointment and cover with gauze dressings if needed.

6.5 Pallor (pale skin)

A pale complexion is often completely normal, but can be a symptom of more serious conditions such as **anaemia, iron deficiency or leukaemia** (See also page 163 on cancer and leukaemia).

> **Seek immediate medical help if you child has the following:**
>
> ### Symptoms
> - Pale mucous membranes
> - Drooping eyelids
> - Pale lips, earlobes and fingernails
> - Lack of energy and listlessness

6.6 Sunburn and sunstroke

Do everything you can to prevent sunburn and overexposure to light before it occurs. **Children's skin is more sensitive to sun**

than that of adults. It is possible for children to get an overdose of sun on their skin even before sunburn or sunstroke is evident.

Be aware of places where the sun's effect is particularly intense: over water, in snow, at high altitudes or in very clear weather. You can develop an awareness of this through your own body, for instance, by concentrating and thinking about when you've been in the sun too long.

Due to thinning of the ozone layer in the stratosphere, the threshold dose for sunburn is reached more quickly today than it used to be, which is a particular concern in the mountains and at high latitudes (southern Australia, New Zealand and northern Europe).

Note that some medicines and remedies can greatly increase the skin's sensitivity to the sun for several weeks, i.e. St John's wort oil and hogweed. Antibiotics and some skin creams for neurodermatitis increase the skin's sensitivity. Read the information that comes with the medicine.

Dermatologists warn against overexposure to sun in childhood and adolescence because it increases the risk of skin cancers later in life.

Sunburn
Symptoms
- Reddening of the skin
- Sensation of heat
- Itching
- Fluid retention (oedema)
- Blistering, if the sunburn is severe
- Later, peeling of skin
- Fever, headache and weakness in severe cases

How you can help
Remedies
- Unless your child is allergic to arnica, apply wet compresses made with Combudoron lotion, ointment or spray or Wala Burn Essence diluted in boiled water. Change the wet compresses frequently or dab the sunburned spots repeatedly.
- Alternatively, quark compresses (see page 297) can be used, but not if your child has eczema or is allergic to cow's milk.
- Calcium Quercus glob. velati or Urtica comp. glob. velati, 5 globules 3–6 times a day, especially for hypersensitivity to sunlight in the spring.

Preventative measures
- Always wear sunhats and T-shirts when outside, even when swimming. Don't let your child run around naked in the sun.
- Never let them fall asleep in the sun.

- It is much healthier to expose children to the sun for shorter periods over several weeks than to expose them for long periods over a shorter timeframe. Short periods outside in the sun in climate conditions to which your children are accustomed are not harmful.
- Sunscreen lotions containing mineral micro-pigments (titanium dioxide, zinc oxide), which are non-allergenic and form a purely physical barrier between the sun and the skin, are recommended over the chemical UV filters commonly used in mainstream sunscreen lotions.
- Sunscreen lotions should not be used on a daily basis as this prevents formation of Vitamin D through the skin.
- Be particularly careful in intense sunlight (at the beach, on water, in mountains or snow) and wear clothing that protects from ultraviolet rays.

Sunstroke
Symptoms
- Headache
- Nausea and vomiting
- Dizziness
- Ringing in the ears
- Fatigue or, in extreme cases, stupor
- Fainting
- Chills and fever as high as 40°C/ 104°F in some cases (usually in conjunction with physical over-exertion under excessively warm conditions and therefore commonly known as 'heatstroke').

How you can help
- Move your child into the shade.
- Give them a cool sponge bath.
- Offer them plenty of fluids to drink.
- Take them to your doctor or to your nearest hospital Accident and Emergency department.
- Take preventative measures as for sunburn (see page 97).

6.7 Dandruff

Causes
- Sensitive scalp skin
- Result of sunburn
- Grass or tree mites
- Cradle cap (see page 114)

How you can help
- Use an anti-dandruff willow-bark shampoo and follow up with a wheatgerm oil conditioner.
- For pronounced dandruff, as in psoriasis, we recommend an application of a heavy-duty moisturiser that is not petroleum-based and then washing it out with a shampoo designed for an itchy or scaly scalp.
- Consult a doctor if no improvement occurs.

6.8 Fungal infections

Worldwide, fungal diseases are on the increase, partly because antibiotics have effectively reduced competition from bacterial infections and partly because the triumph of synthetic fabrics and excessive use of soap and skincare products have contributed to the loss of the skin's protective function against invaders.

In any case, diseases formerly limited to specific occupations with heavy moisture exposure, populations with poor hygiene or exceptionally weakened patients have become familiar (although not a popular topic of conversation) in every family. Our modern lifestyle and clothing preferences – synthetic socks, shoes that are too tight, overly frequent washing or insufficient drying – have become the norm almost everywhere.

Increasing use of antifungal agents has done nothing to reduce the prevalence of fungal skin conditions, demonstrating once again that inefficacy of symptom-suppressing drugs. Genuine healing requires understanding the circumstances under which disease develops and recognising that it will disappear only when these circumstances are eliminated.

Thrush in the mouth and nappy (diaper) area

Thrush usually begins in the mouth and migrates through the digestive tract to the anal area. At this stage, it can be detected in the stools. In severely weakened children or those receiving concurrent treatment with broad-spectrum antibiotics or cortisone asthma treatment, intestinal thrush is extremely persistent. In such cases, the stools smell like yeast.

Symptoms

- *In the mouth:* a fine-textured or coarse network or crumbly white coating, most likely to appear on the insides of the cheeks and on the tongue, but the layer of fungus sometimes extends all the way to the lips.
- A white coating on the tongue without involvement of the mucous membranes of the cheeks, however, is not necessarily a sign of thrush.
- *Around the genital area:* initially dot-like and often oozing nodules, which spread rapidly and merge at least partially, developing thin rings of scales at their edges.

How you can help

- We recommend local treatment with natural remedies. In general, if you are willing to be patient these are successful, even in cases previously treated with antimycotic drugs (usually either nystatin or miconazole) with only temporary success.

- *In the mouth,* the mucous membranes are stabilised by 'brushing' them with swabs dipped in diluted natural mouthwash or mouth balsam (or, in South Africa, Gentian violet 1%), which also removes some of the fungal layer. The fungus does not disappear as quickly as it does under antimycotic treatment, but this is not necessarily a disadvantage, since recurrences are less likely.
- *In the nappy area,* wash the skin first with water and follow up by washing it again with plain (organic) *sunflower seed oil.* (We recommend sunflower oil simply because in the amounts needed it is significantly less expensive than commercial baby oil. Almond or olive oil are good for the skin but more expensive.) Then apply oil that contains an appropriate etheric oil, such as 10% lavender oil, calendula oil or a mixture of the two (note that thyme oil and eucalyptus oil are too irritating). Then apply a protective layer of your regular skin barrier cream.
- Change your baby's nappies as often as possible, including once or twice during the night, to keep contact with dampness as short as possible. Dampness and breakdown products from urine can undo all your therapeutic efforts. We recommend using gauze nappies covered with woollen nappy wraps.
- During this time, sponge-bathe your baby. If you must give them a bath, keep it short so that their skin doesn't soften, which allows the fungus to penetrate deeper.
- Whenever your baby's skin gets wet for any reason, it must be thoroughly dried. You can even use a hairdryer on a low setting, if needed. After drying, apply plenty of oil as outlined above. You can expect to see improvement after 3 or 4 days, although a few new patches may appear. Complete healing, however, takes 2 or 3 weeks.

Athlete's foot (Tinea pedis)
Symptoms
- Crumbly or scaly peeling of the skin, especially between the toes
- Similar but drier peeling, often reddish and forming little blisters on the callused portions of the soles of the feet

How you can help
- As much air and as little water and soap as possible (but as much as necessary, to avoid social isolation due to odour).

101

- After a short footbath in sage or oak bark tea, dry (or blowdry) the affected areas and surrounding skin very thoroughly. Then rub the skin either with an oil that contains an appropriate etheric oil, such as 10% lavender oil, calendula oil or a mixture of the two, or with massage oil that contains only natural etheric oils (no irritating additives).
- Have your child go barefoot or wear open sandals as often as possible.
- Avoid socks made with synthetic fibres or footwear with synthetic linings. Instead, choose wool or cotton socks and change them daily. Make sure your child doesn't wear rubber boots or shoes with synthetic linings for any longer than is absolutely necessary.
- In persistent cases, use a conventional ointment or spray to stop the infection, as the fungus will attack the nails. New, healthy hygiene and clothing practices will ensure that the fungus does not return.

Fungal toenail infection
Causes
- Damage to the nail caused by, for instance, badly fitting shoes, wounds etc., together with a fungal infection between the toes.

Symptoms
- The toenails (very rarely the fingernails) thicken and become yellow-brown, beginning at the edges.

Treatment
- Treatment is long-term, lasting months to years. See a doctor.

6.9 Bacterial skin infections

Erysipelas
- Erysipelas, a bacterial infection that spreads from a small skin injury into the upper layers of the skin and the lymphatic system, is not to be confused with phlegmon. See page 105 for distinguishing characteristics.

Symptoms
- Rash consisting of raised but irregularly bounded bright-red spots that rapidly spread to cover larger areas of hot, reddened skin.
- Swelling that increases with time; sometimes also a bluish discolouration and blister formation.
- Most commonly limited to the foot and lower leg, but may also occur on the face, arms or other parts of the body.

Complications
- If your child has a fever or feels exhausted, have a doctor examine them immediately. An antibiotic treatment will be necessary.

How you can help
- In the early stages, intensive applications of Calendula essence wraps (under a doctor's supervision) can lead to healing.
- During the healing stage, when some pasty swelling remains, applications of Stannum metallicum 0.4%, covered with a cloth, are helpful.
- Internally, Apis mellifica 30X, Lachesis comp. glob. Velati, Myristica sebifera comp. glob. velati or Calendula 4X, may help; the dosage is 5 globules 4–8 times a day.

Impetigo
Impetigo appears mainly in toddlers and in summer. It is very contagious and is difficult to control without antiseptic treatment.

Symptoms
- Isolated itching pustules that rapidly spread
- Pustules usually covered with thick yellow scabs
- Irritated areas of skin (such as under the nose during a cold) are usually affected first
- Scratching spreads the infection

How you can help
- Seek professional help.
- Wash the affected areas of skin with thyme tea several times a day and then apply a drying lotion.
- Alternatively, apply a topical antiseptic like Octenisept several times a day.
- Avoid antibiotic creams if possible, as they increase resistance to antibiotics and there is a danger of developing allergies.
- Children with impetigo should not go to school until a few days after treatment is completed.
- If your child experiences repeated cases of impetigo, consider your environment. For example, if you have a sandpit, old sand may be a possible source of infection.

Alternatives to antibiotics and antiseptics
- In our experience, many bacterial infections can treated by washing with thyme tea, thus avoiding increased resistance to antibiotics and antiseptics.

Folliculitis (infection of the hair follicles)
Causes
- Usually staphylococcus (staph)
- Oily skin
- Increased perspiration

- Inadequate or inappropriate skin hygiene
- Rundown state
- Too much fat in the diet (especially pork and sausage)
- Digestive irregularities with constipation
- Puberty

Symptoms

- Small pustules, sometimes with hairs in the centre

How you can help

- Take steps to reduce the causes outlined above.
- Treat the skin with thyme tea.

Boils, furuncles and carbuncles

Boils or furuncles are pus-forming inflammations that are somewhat larger and sit somewhat deeper in the skin than pimples; very large ones are called carbuncles. If such abscesses occur in the armpits, they are usually inflamed sweat glands.

Symptoms

- Initially as with folliculitis (see above)
- Later, deeper reddening and rough swelling in the area
- A carbuncle is a cluster of interconnected boils; the reddened, swollen area surrounds all of them.

Complications

- Open, suppurative ulcerations and necrotic tissue may develop if treatment is delayed and the wound-healing process is disrupted.

How you can help
Remedies

- *In the early stages*, we have had success with Calendula–Echinacea ointment wraps, using Calcea ointment (Wala Calcea Wund- und Heilcreme), for example.
- *In acute cases*: echinacea juice, 1 teaspoon 3 times a day; Calendula 4X, 5–10 globules 5–8 times a day; Hepar sulfuris 6X, 5–10 globules 5–8 times a day.
- *An abscess that has come to a head* usually needs to be lanced by a doctor.
- If your child has *several boils at the same time or if they appear repeatedly* (more likely in toddlers and school-age children than in infants), they should be tested for diabetes. Once this has been done, constitutional treatment (see page 248) may alleviate or cure the problem. This treatment is carried out for at least 4–6 weeks and can be continued, if needed, for 2 months longer or repeated after a 4-week break. We recommend: echinacea juice, 1 teaspoon twice a day;

Calendula 4X, 5–10 globules 3 times a day; and Hepar sulfuris 6X, 5–10 globules 3 times a day.

Phlegmon

This is an inflammation of the tissue. Unlike with boils and carbuncles, where the body builds up a protective wall to contain the pus, with phlegmon no barrier forms to contain the pus.

Symptoms

In contrast to Erysipelas (see page 102):

- All layers of tissue can be affected
- The pus-forming and painful inflammation is more diffuse but spreads faster
- Generally the child feels worse
- Fever occurs sooner and more often

How you can help

- Phlegmon seldom occurs, but requires prompt treatment and hospitalisation.

Infections of the hand

Cracks or wounds on the fingers or on the palm of the hand give easy access to deeper layers of skin and lead to acute pus-forming infections. Minor nail-bed infections (whitlows) develop easily in young infants, either spontaneously or because their fingernails are cut too soon. An infection of this type usually heals well when kept covered in medicated ointment, but get your doctor to take a look at it if the inflammation spreads to encompass the entire first joint of the finger.

Do not use an adhesive bandage or tape on infants: it might cut off circulation in a finger or your baby might choke on it if it comes off. Even for older children, adhesive bandages are usually not the most effective way to cover infected spots.

If your child has a progressive, throbbing infection on a finger, consult a doctor as soon as possible. Even a day's delay can cause permanent damage or even, in severe cases, the loss of the finger.

Take the same precaution if there is an infection where the nail and skin meet at the side or the base of a fingernail (paronchia).

Symptoms

- Redness surrounding a fingernail or toenail
- Swelling, sensitivity to pressure
- Throbbing pain
- Pus formation
- Fever and chills, if complications develop

How you can help

- Apply a dollop of medicated ointment to the affected finger and then cover all the fingers with a piece of gauze fastened at the wrist. Cover the gauze with a mitten-like sack knotted loosely at the wrist. Change the entire bandage once or twice a day.

- At every change of bandage you can bathe the hand in thyme tea.
- Surgical treatment becomes necessary if the inflammation spreads.

Remedies

- Internally, either Myristica sebifera comp. glob. velati, 5 globules 4–6 times a day, or Calendula 4X, 5 globules 4–6 times a day.

Blood poisoning

Blood poisoning is more correctly described as purulent inflammation of the lymph vessels (lymphangitis). It usually appears after a minor injury that may even be overlooked, through bacteria entering the tissue. Medical attention is required.

Seek medical attention if:

Symptoms

- Red stripes appear suddenly, running up or down the inside of an arm or leg, for example.
- Lymph nodes in the armpit or groin quickly swell and become painful.
- Possibly fever.

How you can help

- Compresses moistened with a Calendula essence.
- The affected limb is immobilised with a splint.
- A tetanus booster shot is often recommended.
- Special caution is needed if your child also has a fever; an antibiotic may be necessary.
- The bacteria's point of entry must be cleaned up.

Remedies

- In addition, we recommend Erysidoron 1 (Apis 3X and Belladonna 3X), up to 5 drops in a little water every hour (it's best to hold it in the mouth for a bit before swallowing), or Myristica sebifera comp. glob. velati, 5 globules 6–8 times a day, allowed to dissolve slowly in the mouth.

6.10 Viral skin infections

Fever blisters (cold sores, herpes simplex)

Fever blisters are caused by the same virus as mouth ulcers (see page 142).

Symptoms

- Slightly itchy small blisters filled with a clear liquid

- Blisters do not contain pus
- Usually only on the lips

How you can help

- Treat with a very thin coating of drying cream, for instance a soft zinc paste (if nothing else is to hand, any toothpaste will help).
- Alternatively, treat with an anti-inflammatory cream, e.g. 1.0 g acetylsalicyl acid, 14.0 g Vaseline.
- Labimint Acute Lip Care (Dr Hauschka) can also help; like lip balms with echinacea, it is also good for prevention.
- LomaHerpan Creme with lemon balm extract can also relieve symptoms.
- **If there is suspicion of infection in early infancy, see your doctor urgently to check for encephalitis.**

Prevention

- If you have herpes, strictly avoid any intimate contact that might transmit the virus to your baby. Disinfect your hands and do not kiss your baby or snuggle with them. If you are nursing, you must wear a face mask!

Warts

Warts are benign growths on the skin. Because they are triggered by viruses, they are contagious and their development is dependent on your immune status. They tend to occur more frequently in puberty, for example, when resistance is low and physical contact with others increases.

There are eight different types of warts, with the following commonly occurring in children and adolescents: juvenile warts, flat warts, plantar warts, filiform warts, mosaic warts, molluscum contagiosum (or water warts), common warts and genital warts, which appear only after sexual intercourse and in the genital area.

Warts are transmitted by smear infection and minor injuries; transmission of molluscum contagiosum is especially common in swimming pools.

Symptoms

- Raised warts on the fingers are usually common warts.
- Flat but sometimes deep-seated and heavily callused warts on the foot are often plantar warts or juvenile warts, which can also appear on all other parts of the body but are less conspicuous there.
- Molluscum contagiosum is characterised by multiple firm, pinhead-sized keratinous nodules with central openings. They generally develop on more delicate areas of skin.

How you can help
Remedies
- Mosts warts respond to ointment containing bismuth and antimony, applied twice daily for 1–3 months.
- Apply thuja or tea tree oil once or twice daily, less often if reddening occurs.
- Dab with the fresh sap of greater celandine (*Chelidonium majus*).
- Corn plasters are not helpful, but for plantar warts it may be necessary to treat the callus so the active ingredients can get through to the underlying layers.
- Internally, to stimulate the immune system, for 4–6 weeks: Thuja e summitatibus 4X glob. velati, 5–10 globules 3 times a day; echinacae juice, ½–1 teaspoon 3 times a day.
- Surgical removal or cryotherapy is often attempted, but scraping out molluscum contagiosum often spreads the infection and causes relapses. Because we have had good success with the above-mentioned therapies, surgical removal is generally not necessary.

Viral exanthemas
An exanthema is a rash accompanying a disease or fever. Many non-specific rashes are caused by viruses. Treatment that specifically targets the rash is seldom necessary. See Chapter 7 on childhood diseases (page 127) for more information on the most common viral exanthemas.

6.11 Insect bites and skin parasites

Bee and wasp stings
If your child is allergic to bee stings or if the stinger hits a blood vessel, a serious systemic reaction can develop, like swelling of the mucous membranes, breathing or circulatory difficulties, or even an allergic (anaphylactic) shock (see page 18). **Take your child to a doctor immediately, or call emergency services if they experience breathing and circulatory difficulties.**

How you can help
- Immediately remove the stinger to avoid more poison seeping out, by scraping across it with a flat edged object (e.g. a credit card).
- Do not squeeze the stinger out, as this can make more poison enter the tissue.
- Do not suck the wound and spit out the poison, as the poison can be absorbed through tiny wounds in the gum of the helper, possibly causing fresh problems.

- If available, press a freshly cut onion on the sting.
- Alternatively, use moist compresses made with diluted nettle / arnica extract (Combudoron).
- Apis mellifica 30X, 5 globules 3–6 times daily.

Mosquito bites
How you can help
- Dab the bites with saliva or water, then spread a little soap over the area. The itching will immediately lessen.
- If the itching is severe, use Combudoron gel or lotion that contains a nettle / arnica extract.

Prevention
- Watery emulsions of etheric oils (Zedan insect repellent etc.) are available from your pharmacy or natural health store and will repel insects for several hours.
- In areas where mosquitoes are numerous at night, it is a good idea to hang mosquito netting over the bed, particularly for infants and toddlers.

Scabies
Causes
- Scabies is caused by mites.

Symptoms
- Inflamed areas of skin
- The parasites themselves are almost never seen

- Other members of the family are usually affected as well
- Eczema may persist for weeks if caused by traces of mite excrement
- It is possible to mistake scabies for chronic endogenous eczema (see page 116)

How you can help
- Clothing must be boiled, dry-cleaned or hung outside for 4 days.
- Your doctor will prescribe medication.
- Combudoron gel or essence can relieve an itchy rash.
- Scabies must be distinguished from the bites of grass mites, which usually move from grasses to humans only briefly, sucking blood and dropping off again. Grass mite bites cause a very itchy rash that disappears on its own after about 10 days. Again, Combudoron is helpful.

Flea bites
- Fleas may migrate from domestic or wild animals to humans.

Symptoms
- Bites arranged in rows (along the waistband, for example).
- Inflammatory changes (increased swelling, reddening and fluid build-up) may occasionally develop.

How you can help

- Apply Combudoron gel or essence.
- If a secondary infection develops, dab the affected spots with diluted Calendula essence.
- Fill your bath with water and shake out used clothing and bedding over it.
- For both acute flea infestation and just a few fleas, a diatomaceous earth product (made up of microscopic bodies of fossilised phyto-plankton) will kill the insects by drying them out. It is harmless to humans and animals.
- For persistent infestations with larvae present, a non-toxic product that works on both larvae and adults, such Neudorff's Neudo Antifloh, may be needed.

Head lice (nits)

These are very common and tiresome in kindergartens and schools. They are not a sign of inadequate hygiene and do not carry any contagious illnesses.

Symptoms

- Itchy scalp
- Head lice are found approximately 1 cm (½ inch) above the scalp
- Lice of different sizes (developmental stages) may be visible

How you can help

- The current recommendation is to use an oily substance. These products coat the lice with oil and kill them by clogging their respiratory passages. The lice and eggs can then be washed out.
- Remove as many lice and eggs as possible, either with an aluminum comb (which can hurt) or by cutting out individual hairs that still have lice on them. Combing should be done daily until all lice and eggs have been removed. Clean the comb between strokes.
- Treat the entire family.
- Search every family member for head lice and eggs. They are found approximately 1 cm (½ inch) above the scalp. If they are more than 3 cm (1 inch) up, you can be certain that they are dead.
- An alternative is 30 minutes of treatment with hot air, such as a soft bonnet hair dryer, but be careful to avoid burns.
- According to recent studies, the formerly recommended natural extracts of pyrethrum and neem are no longer adequately effective, due to increased resistance, and may cause allergies.
- We cannot recommend the use of other chemical products for initial treatment due to their toxicity.
- Clothing, bed linen and soft toys do not need to be treated, merely

kept away from people for 24 hours, as head lice will become immobile after this time without regular blood-sucking. After 55 hours they will all have died. Eggs are only deposited in hair.

Further measures

Do not let embarrassment prevent you from informing your child's teacher and other parents as soon as you discover a lice infestation, and request that they check for any further cases. Full disclosure is the only way to prevent both the spread of lice and reinfestations. Your children (although no longer contagious themselves) may easily bring a louse home from school or kindergarten again the very next day. That is why it is important to know that lice are not a sign of inadequate hygiene and therefore no cause for embarrassment.

Make sure you are aware of any local regulations excluding louse-infested individuals from school or public events. Children should return to school only when no more nits can be found on their heads. (They may still have a few empty or dead nits in their hair even after they are completely free of lice, but without examining the nits under a microscope, you will not be able to tell whether they are old or new ones.)

Tick bites

See page 152 and Lyme disease, Section 7.

6.12 Allergic and toxic skin reactions

The many different chemicals found in cleaning supplies, laundry softeners, hand creams, cosmetics, textile treatments etc. have produced a multitude of allergic skin reactions. Of course, such reactions can also be triggered by natural materials like plant extracts or metals.

Allergic contact dermatitis

Walking or working in the open can sometimes lead to inadvertent contact with plants of all kinds that cause skin reactions and rashes. In some areas, contact with poison ivy can cause severe itching and redness of the skin. Other plants that give contact dermatitis are yarrow, primula, sumac and poison oak. In North America, cow parsnip, a *Heracleum* species, causes photo-dermatitis, a rash very similar to a burn, with reddening and blistering of the skin. Treatment is the same as for sunburn. Children should be taught to recognise these plants in their locality and avoid contact if possible.

Allergic reactions

Allergic reactions can appear over the whole body, on the skin or mucous membranes, in the bronchi, or as a circulatory reaction, as the immune system overreacts (see also *Allergic (anaphylactic) shock,* page 18). Allergies appear whatever the quantity of trigger chemical, but only in those people who have allergies.

Their manifestations vary so greatly that we might almost say that there is no skin ailment that cannot be mimicked by an allergic episode. If an allergy is suspected, experiment with avoiding specific substances to see if the symptoms recede.

Certain skin allergies, some of which cause hives, are reactions to medications such as antibiotics and sulfonamides; see Hives (Urticaria) below.

How you can help

- Baths containing horsetail (equisetum) tea (see page 313); if blisters are present, also add sage tea.
- In acute cases, take 5 Urtica comp. globules or Calcium quercus globules hourly.
- In the longer term, take a pinch Quarz12X trit. 3 times daily.
- Depending on the overall allergic picture, constitutional remedies (see page 248) may be used to stimulate liver or kidney activity or other metabolic functions. Consult your doctor.

Hives (urticaria)
Causes
- In most cases the cause is unknown.
- Possible overreaction to foods, medicines, insecticides, heat, cold or pressure on the skin.
- Side effect of immunological processes, for instance viral infections with diarrhoea or other metabolic disturbances.
- Factors like stress.
- Hard cheese and cocoa exacerbate hives, because of their histamine content.

Symptoms
- Swollen areas that are either pale against a red background or reddened against a background of normal skin, similar to rashes cause by nettles or horsefly bites.
- Irregularly distributed and highly irregular in shape.
- Severe itching. Patients tend to rub the spots rather than scratch them.
- Duration ranges from hours to weeks.
- Chronic hives are rare; this requires constitutional treatment by a doctor.

Complications

- In severe cases, swelling of the face and the mucous membranes of the mouth, throat and larynx (Quincke's oedema) may occur. **Seek immediate medical attention in such cases, since they can lead to life-threatening respiratory distress.**

How you can help

- Avoid triggers.
- Consider maintaining a diet low in histamine content.
- A powder that soothes itching can be helpful in milder cases.
- Ammi visnaga tincture 1X, up to 5 drops every hour in a little water.
- **Seek medical attention immediately if your child feels generally unwell or develops complications.**

Photodermatitis

Photodermatitis is a light-activated allergic reaction brought about by the combination of sun exposure and contact (often unnoticed) with certain plants in the Umbelliferae family, such as wild parsnip or giant hogweed or with dictamnus (also known as burning bush).

Symptoms

- Burn-like reddening and blistering of the skin after a walk or working in the garden
- Can persist for several weeks
- Dark discolouration of the skin post-healing

How you can help

- As for sunburn (see page 97).
- Keep the affected areas covered with clothing.

Strophulus (Simple acute prurigo)

Causes

- For the most part, the causes are unknown, although some cases can be traced to heightened reactions to mites or flea bites.

Symptoms

- Reddish or pale knot-like bumps on the skin, a few millimeters in diameter
- Blistering is possible
- Localised on the trunk and the extensor sides of the extremities

How you can help

- First-aid measures are the same as for allergic reactions and hives (see opposite page).
- Apply Combudoron gel.

6.13 Chronic allergic skin infections

Seborrhoeic dermatitis

Seborrhoeic dermatitis, which has no common name in English, is an inflammatory skin disease caused by an irregular flow of sebum. In this condition, the skin's vegetative activity is too strong, resulting in increased fat production and the development of greasy scales. It is generally due to hormonal changes after birth and often disappears by the time your baby is 4 months old.

It is not always easy for doctors to distinguish seborrhoeic dermatitis from fungal infections, especially since fungal infection or suppuration may occur secondarily, and it is also often confused with cradle cap (see below).

Symptoms
- Greasy, soft, yellowish-brown scales on skin that is only slightly reddened, if at all
- Generally limited to the scalp
- However, it can appear in the face, in folds of the skin or in the nappy area and in rare cases over the entire body
- Usually appears about a week after birth
- Little or no itching

How you can help
- Almond oil baths are a suitable treatment: 1 teaspoon almond oil in 250 ml/1 US cup of milk, mixed well into the bathwater.
- Treat affected areas with almond oil, olive oil or sage oil (maximum 5%).
- *Important:* **Do not use peanut oil instead of almond oil.**

Cradle cap

Cradle cap is often confused with seborrhoeic dermatitis of the scalp (see above). It is an early form of (and usually transitions into) chronic atopic dermatitis.

Symptoms
- Hard scales and crusting of skin that may be significantly reddened, oozing or scratched raw
- Usually appears after the age of 3 months
- Itching may be severe
- General well-being is sometimes impacted

How you can help
- If *itching*, dab the affected areas with horsetail tea.
- If *severe oozing* is present, dab with black tea.
- If a *superinfection develops* (with oozing, pustules and inflamed yellowish crusting), dab with thyme tea.
- When eczema and itching occur together, a cool ointment helps. Ask your pharmacist to prepare

this formula for you: 70g aqueous decoction of *Equisetum arvense* and 10g pure urea in 200g anhydrous eucerin. Apply a thin layer of this ointment several times a day.
- It also helps to apply olive oil, followed by washing with a gentle anti-dandruff shampoo.
- To avoid injuring the scalp, wait until the scales start to flake off by themselves before removing them gently with a comb. Premature removal can encourage infection and the flaking will quickly return.

Psoriasis

Psoriasis is one of the exanthemas that run in families. It was formerly thought to have nothing to do with neurodermatitis, but now we know that the transition from neurodermatitis to psoriasis is more common than previously believed. Although the causes of psoriasis have not yet been definitively explained, autoimmune factors are suspected.

Symptoms
- Manifests in many different forms, often affecting more than just the scalp
- Typically appears as clearly defined red patches of slightly raised skin covered with large silvery scales
- Usually at joints, like elbows or knees, or on the scalp, in the face or on the chest
- Pitted and thickened nails
- Often itches
- Rare in young children, and in school children more common than neurodermatitis
- May affect joints

How you can help
- Avoid triggers such as injuries, and mechanical irritation like tattoos, cold and stress.
- Good nourishment is important: avoid animal fats, pork, hot spices and too many sweets, particularly food additives (colouring or flavourings).
- Sunlight is beneficial.
- Seawater helps: an occasional evening bath with sea salt helps, as do vacations by the sea.
- Extra attention to skincare is important. We recommend aloe vera or mallow body lotion.
- For medications, a great variety of constitutional remedies are possible, some of which are the same as for neurodermatitis (see page 116). Cichorium/Pancreas comp. glob. velati have sometimes yielded interesting successes for us.

6.14 Chronic endogenous eczema, atopic dermatitis or neurodermatitis

These three names refer to the same condition, namely, constitutional susceptibility to *eczema*. There are genetic connections to hay fever and asthma, i.e. there is a hereditary predisposition to eczema. However, the susceptibility can arise anew.

This syndrome has become increasingly common in recent decades. Contributing factors include environmental pollutants and food allergens as well as general changes in lifestyles and human habits (see page 125).

Causes
- Half of all children with this condition have a family history of eczema.
- Some have food or milk allergies or other allergic reactions to dust mites, pollen, cleaning products etc.
- Look out for non-specific factors like stress, heat or change in weather.

Symptoms
- The most obvious symptom is itching, often so severe that children scratch themselves bloody.
- In infants, the skin of the head and shoulders is affected; in pre-schoolers, the folds of the large joints and the backs of the hands; and in older children, the torso and limbs
- The skin is usually uniformly dry.
- The rash typically consists of firm, itching nodules, which may appear in groups, forming raised patches.
- The rash may ooze or look raw; if scratched, it may be covered with crusty scabs.
- Apart from strong itching, it is typical that the skin's appearance can change quickly: for instance, in the morning the skin may be raw and open, but by the afternoon looks much better; on the following day it is almost healed, but overnight opens again.

How you can help
- Carefully observe changes in the skin. It may help to keep a diary over several weeks, noting weather, stress factors, food etc. This can be helpful when discussing with your doctor what the best treatment is or whether further tests are necessary.
- Keep the itching areas of skin completely covered with cotton underwear or with a one-piece coverall that also encloses the hands. You can make this yourself by adapting the size of the pattern on page 315. Your child

will love this outfit because you made it! Embroider it with sun, moon and stars (using soft cotton thread to avoid itching) or paint friendly little faces on the hands. Your child will play with their 'puppets' for hours and will not be able to scratch.

- It's important for parents to remain as calm and objective as possible. Often, a child's severe itching tests the strength of the entire family. Parents can find themselves on the verge of despair and at the end of their tether because they never get a good night's sleep. A child with eczema soon learns to use scratching as a way to get what they want, refusing to sleep in their own bed and always demanding the opposite of what anyone else wants. Once the family pet, your child can soon become the family tyrant. The only way to prevent this is to treat a child with eczema as 'normally' as possible. Implement the treatments listed above as matter-of-factly as you can and then return to your daily routine without showering your child with further attention.
- Take particular care with chickenpox and chronic eczema. Chickenpox are often more severe, and after the attack of chickenpox the eczema can become markedly better, but

unfortunately in as many cases it becomes markedly worse. A chickenpox vaccination may be considered but has no beneficial effect on the neurodermatitis.

- A harmless herpes infection can also be much more severe with chronic eczema.

Psychological considerations

The skin is an organ that protects our contact with the outer world. On the one hand, the dry skin of an eczema patient seems less alive and more of a barrier than normal; on the other hand, it reacts with greater sensitivity and exudative (oozing) eczema is too alive and open.

You can help your child shift their emotional focus from their body to their surroundings not only by providing a protective covering of topical medications (ointments or compresses) and suitable clothing but also by fostering their interest in what is going on around them. If you also allow them to experience clear limits (that is, if you as parents are sure of what you want and of what needs to be done at the moment), their personality will grow stronger and they will be able to redefine their relationship to the world. This approach has positive effects on the illness and goes a long way towards alleviating skin symptoms.

Feeding a baby with neurodermatitis

Ideally, your baby should be exclusively breastfed for a minimum of 4 months. Parsnips or pumpkin are appropriate first solid foods.

To ensure that new foods are tolerated, always try out only one new food at a time, keeping in mind there may be a delay of as long as 72 hours before skin reactions appear.

We have had positive experiences in introducing solid foods while babies are still nursing, which we recommend especially when introducing less well-tolerated foods, such as cow's milk.

Citrus fruits, even ingested second-hand in breast milk, always exacerbate eczema. Organic and especially Demeter-certified products are tolerated significantly better than conventional products.

The chart below gives an overview of how well-selected individual foods are tolerated.

If over a period of days your baby reacts with only mild eczema to foods containing cow's milk, it is an individual decision whether to tolerate these skin symptoms and continue to feed your baby cow's milk in the form of mild yoghurt, for example, or to switch to expensive mare's or goat's milk. This also applies when the infant reacts to the nursing mother's milk consumption.

We advise against constantly experimenting with changes in your baby's staple foods. In most cases these are the wrong suspects and can lead to an ever-growing spiral of things to avoid, which causes unnecessary stress and exacerbates the condition.

Very well tolerated	Less well tolerated	Often not tolerated
Parsnips	Kohlrabi	Tomatoes, ketchup
Pumpkin	Beets	Carrots (except Demeter carrots, which are well tolerated)
Courgettes/zucchini	Oats	Peppers
Chard	Rice	Wheat
Potatoes	Corn	Soya
Quinoa	Barley	Cow's milk

Buckwheat	Spelt	Eggs
Millet	Goat's milk	Pork
Amaranth	Yoghurt	Sausage
Veal	Cream, cheese	Nuts (hazelnuts, cashews, peanuts)
Lamb	Fish	Citrus fruits
Pears	Beef	Strawberries
Apples	Almonds, almond butter	Kiwi fruit
Olive oil and safflower	Butter	Spicy foods
	Honey	Chocolate
	Maple syrup	Refined sugar

Tolerability of individual foods

If in the first months there is a reasonable suspicion of allergy to some foodstuff, cut it out for 4 weeks and then give it again, unless the reaction was quite unequivocal or went beyond symptoms of the skin. Breastfeeding mothers should follow the same procedure if they think something they are eating causes their baby's allergy. If this experiment confirms your suspicions, then go to your doctor, who can confirm this either with a blood test or a provocation.

If the allergy is proven, avoid this food for a year, but then try it again. After a severe allergic reaction with systemic symptoms or even anaphylactic shock, your baby should be hospitalised while foods are retested. Food allergies often disappear after some months, unlike those caused by pollen, animal dander or dust mites.

Distinguish allergies (see page 111) from toxic reactions. They are signs of irritation that everyone has to a greater or lesser extent; the sensitive skin of someone suffering from chronic eczema will show a stronger reaction, so it is best to avoid these substances. Examples are etheric oils (citrus oils, eucalyptus oils), spices and food additives (phosphates and

119

enhancers). We are often unaware of these additives; for instance, almost all non-organic chocolate contains several additives.

You can expect diet-related eczema to improve spontaneously and significantly in your child's second year of life. Nonetheless, many eczema patients remain sensitive to citrus fruits and other acidic foods, as well as nuts and sometimes fish and eggs. Fermented milk products are often tolerated even when fresh milk still triggers eczema. Honey and sweets may make eczema symptoms worse, but true allergic reactions are not involved in this case. Therefore sweet things in moderation will not harm your child.

Skincare

We do not recommend cortisone ointments and use them only when either the parents or the child cannot afford the extra time required for alternative therapies, or for short-term respite in especially desperate situations involving severe itching and too many sleepless nights.

How you can help

The suggestions that follow are intended as aids in the period before individualised treatment is agreed with your doctor.

Severely oozing

- Apply wet, cool compresses made with black tea (2 teaspoons to 1 litre/quart, steep for 15 minutes).

Severely inflamed oozing

- Dab the affected areas with a damp cloth.
- Daily sponge baths with thyme tea (2 teaspoons per litre/quart, steep for 10 minutes).
- Apply Pekur Spezialpflegecreme thinly to the inflamed spots once a day.

Acute itching

- Dab the areas with horsetail tea (1 heaped tablespoon soaked for 12 hours, if possible, in 1 litre/quart of cold water, then boiled for 15 minutes).
- For skincare, we recommend once daily use of a gentle natural product such as Pekur Intensivpflegelotion, Pekur Spezialpflegecreme or Halicar crème, which contains a Cardiospermum extract, the 'homeopathic cortisone'.

Subacute redness

- Use a lotion or non-greasy ointment such as Pekur Basishautpflegecreme Level 1 to 3 or Halicar Crème.
- Give your baby a once-weekly sponge bath with Viola tricolour

tea (2 teaspoons per litre/quart, steeped for 10 minutes).

Chronic redness

- Use a mild skin cream such as Pekur Basishautpflegecreme Level 4 to 6 or Halicar Crème.
- Give your baby a once-weekly sponge bath with Viola tricolour tea (2 teaspoons per litre/quart, steeped for 10 minutes).

Chronically dry, calloused

- Apply a greasy ointment such as 'cool ointment' (70g aqueous decoction of Equisetum arvense and 10g pure urea in 200g anhydrous eucerin), Imlan Crème or Pekur Intensivpflegecreme.
- Give your baby a weekly sponge bath with Viola tricolour tea (see above).

Medical Treatment

We recommend a constitutional treatment (see page 248) prescribed by an experienced family doctor or paediatrician. In our experience, quartz or silica compounds are suitable basic remedies for the skin and sensory organs.

- Quartz 20X trituration, 1 pea-sized portion 3 times a day, when the senses are very alert and overstimulated.
- Quartz 6X trituration, 1 pea-sized portion 3 times a day, to support the recovery in the skin's sensory organ.
- Equisetum arvense Silicea cultum Rh 3X, 5–10 drops 3 times a day to 'enliven' the skin.
- Nontronite (Ferrum silicicum) 6X trituration, 1 pea-sized portion 3 times a day, for boundary strengthening.

It is also very important, however, to support and regulate specific metabolic functions, which depending on your child's constitution may result in significant relief of symptoms, especially itching. Finding the right treatment for each individual child and their particular acute problem takes time and close medical supervision. For example, the following steps can aid in metabolic regulation and detoxification:

- Optimising the intestinal flora, especially by supplementing with lactobacteria, can achieve positive effects.
- Cichorium e planta tota 5% glob. velati, 5–10 globules 3–6 times a day for multiple thin, acidic stools. *Caution:* may cause constipation in too high a dose.
- Hepatodoron, 1–2 tablets in the evening, to strengthen liver function.
- Cichorium Stanno cultum Rh 3X Dil., 5 drops daily to support absorption of nutrients from the intestines.

- Lycopodium e planta tota 12X, 3 globules 4–8 times a day, for flatulence.
- Equisetum arvense Silicea cultum Rh 3X, 5 drops 3 times a day, to strengthen kidney function.

Examples of medications to *relieve itching* include:

- Calcium Quercus glob. velati, up to 3 globules per hour.
- Urtica comp. glob. velati, 5 globules 3-6 times a day.
- Bryophyllum 5X/Conchae 7X, 1 ampoule orally, at night.
- Bryophyllum 50% powder, ½ teaspoon once or twice daily, in the evening or at night.
- Arsenicum album 12X, 5 globules in the evening.

Dyshidrotic eczema (pompholyx)

Dyshidrotic eczema is an unspecific eczema, that is a kind of 'sensitive skin'. Frequently it is found in children or teenagers who still have a mild form of, or previously had, neurodermatitis.

Causes

- Sweat
- Stress
- Some leather-tanning materials
- Non-leather shoes
- Seawater
- Contact allergies, e.g. chrome, nickel, latex

Symptoms

- First shows small blisters on the edges of the palms of the hand and soles of feet
- Later, moist parts on palms, between fingers and on soles
- Itching
- In bad cases, the palms or soles have open wounds
- More common in winter and in summer

How you can help

- Give foot and hand baths in a decoction of old oak leaves. Gather the last brown leaves from the trees in early spring and pour boiling water over them. Let them soak for 5–10 minutes before removing the leaves. Let the water cool and then bathe feet or hands for about 10 minutes.
- Foot and hand baths with decoction of sage leaves.
- Give your child a cup of sage tea in the mornings.
- Rub on a little cream (for instance, Nivea) and bandage. The ointment must not contain any lanolin.
- Give 5–10 drops of Ammi visnage 1X in some water 3–6 times daily.

6.15 Allergic sensitivity

Allergies are the result of a complex disturbance in the balance of the immune system. The immune system is affected by stress, over-sensitivity to toxic influences and sensory over-alertness and over-stimulation, all of which weaken the body and its ability to separate itself from the environment. Thus treatment of allergies is based on supporting boundary demarcation and reducing sensitivity. Achieving this is a challenge.

Immune response as a learning process

There is a worldwide increase in people suffering from active or atopic allergies. The most common allergic diseases of childhood are chronic eczema (see page 116), asthma (see page 76) and hayfever (see page 80).

The healthy body protects and defends its identity by equipping all of its organ surfaces and all surfaces in contact with the outer world (skin, lungs, intestines) with protective functions. We call the sum total of all these normal protective functions 'the immune system'. But when these functions get out of balance and 'overreact'

to specific substances, the result is allergic symptoms.

When allergens (allergy-triggering foreign substances) are ingested (in food or medications), or inhaled or touched (certain plants or animal hair), the body's endogenous defences are strongly activated. Instead of learning to deal with certain substances, the body overreacts to resist them. This resistance causes skin rashes, itching, swelling of the mucous membranes, diarrhoea or other symptoms. Specific (and often non-specific) antibodies to these allergens are formed in the blood or on cell surfaces. Since the bloodstream carries antibodies throughout the body, merely touching an allergy-triggering food with one hand may be enough to cause swollen lips and a red face.

Antibody formation is the basis of immunity. With regard to infectious diseases, it is highly desirable. It often occurs unnoticed, in 'silent' or subclinical infections. In allergies, however, it becomes a problem. Excessive antibody production interacts with other processes to produce allergic symptoms. In some cases, however, allergy-prone bodies do learn to deal with allergens over a number of years. Therefore we are especially concerned to encourage use of the suggestions that follow to support the body in its capacity to change and willingness to learn.

Learning as a preventative measure against allergies

Epigenetic research in the last thirty years has confirmed that an individual's genetic potential is an open system that is not only capable of lifelong learning but can also be stimulated from both sides: by the outer world on the one hand and by the inner world of thoughts and feelings on the other. For this reason, a good balance between educational and remedial measures strengthens the immune system.

One of Rudolf Steiner's most pertinent discoveries was that the body's self-healing forces (and thus also immunoregulation) are related to the activity of thinking. Steiner describes the etheric 'life' body not only as the vehicle of self-regulation and healing but also as the vehicle of a person's thought processes (see page 237). Therefore immunological functions depend not only on heredity but also on your child's own capacity for learning and enthusiasm, as well as on the lifestyle (in the broadest sense) cultivated at home and in school.

Good conventional treatment of chronic allergies is based on more than simply administering medications. Patient education and individualised advice, up to and including educational issues (for example, how can a child who is allergic to hay participate in a hands-on farming block), have become increasingly important.

In addition, the development of immunocompetence can be enhanced if children enjoy learning from the very beginning. Joy in learning and the willingness to see ever-new aspects of old, familiar things and to process negative experiences in positive ways are much easier for children to learn if these attitudes are modelled at home and practised in kindergarten and at school.

This is important because it supports the development of healthy self-awareness and a sense of identity and helps children process what they encounter. Aaron Antonovsky's 'sense of coherence' is also a decisive factor in achieving and maintaining stable good health: when children experience the world as 'coherent' understandable, meaningful and manageable they become psychologically 'immune', i.e. resilient and less easily injured.

In years to come, lifestyle research based on the model of salutogenesis (see page 236) will increase our understanding of 'diseases of civilisation', such as atopic allergy. Attentive self-observation, however, can already tell us which circumstances make us feel better and which ones intensify healthy sensitivity to the point of over-re-activity and self-destructive vul-nerability. Individuals alive today are already the third generation to experience the challenges posed by declining values, fear of life, doubt in the meaning of human exist-ence and horror in the face of mass misery and terrorism. Initially, all of these concerns and questions are depressing and weaken healthy immune responses. In the longer term, however, coping in positive ways, self-acceptance and creative cultural involvement counteract allergic sensitivity as effectively as loss of positivity and sense of pur-pose promote it.

Causes

- The widespread use of many new substances in the environ-ment and in food and clothing.
- Excessive hygiene and city chil-dren's lack of exposure to plant and animal allergens.
- Increasing numbers of one-child families.
- Too short a time (less than 4 months) breastfeeding, or not breastfeeding (see page 190).
- Active ingredients and additives in early, multiple vaccinations (see Chapter 14).

- Conventional agricultural prac-tices and industrial processing of foods.
- Inappropriate treatment of fevers, especially the regular use of paracetamol/acetaminophen.
- Antibiotic use in medical treat-ment and in conventional agri-cultural practices.
- Haste and stress.
- Loss of identity and the feeling of not being 'accepted'.

How you can help

- A change of climate of at least 4 weeks may force the body to change, adapt and generally become more flexible.
- Allow your child to experience fever: high fevers accompany-ing childhood illnesses place heavy demands on the entire immune system and may make it stronger and more func-tional.
- Eat healthy, simple food.
- Live or spend time in the coun-tryside (a farm is ideal).
- Accept your children and let them know that they are 'all right just the way they are'.
- Promote your child's creativity, for example, through a limited number of toys that permit many different experiences.
- Support their attentiveness by cultivating sensory impressions (see page 202).

- Create a sense of security and trust through a regular, rhythmical daily routine.
- Set clear limits.
- Be decisive in your actions, and accompany this with loving willingness to adapt to, and take direction from, life's concrete situations.
- Take the constructive attitude that we can learn from life's hidden dangers and that we have the outer and inner resources to cope with them.

7. Infectious Childhood Illnesses

Our level of trust in children's own healing forces depends on what we experience in dealing with their first few infections. We all know that we cannot expect childhood to be free of tests such as infections, spiking fevers and illnesses, yet parents faced with their child's first illness will be uncertain and anxious. Suddenly, your child is different, whether sensitive, irritable and cranky or unusually serious, quiet and hot with fever. To enable parents to deal with these situations, it helps to recognise these childhood illnesses and to see them not simply as problems but also as factors contributing to the development of a more stable state of health later in life.

Infectious diseases

In contrast to the allergic illnesses described in Chapter 6, each infectious disease leads to recovery through a surprisingly regular, predictable series of interactions between 'offensive' and 'defensive' processes. Because of this predictability, these infections are also called 'self-limiting' diseases. Their main visible symptoms (fever, rashes, swollen lymph nodes or vomiting) are usually signs of the body's struggle to overcome the infection. They are part and parcel of the body's response to the illness, and they pave the way for overcoming it, i.e. for achieving a new state of equilibrium on a higher level of immunity. This difference between infectious and allergic illnesses may explain why the latter sometimes improve after young patients undergo classic children's illnesses and why asthma is less prevalent in parts of the world where small children experience many infections.

Many of today's adults still owe the strength and flexibility of their immune systems to the fact that as children they were allowed to learn to cope with germs, i.e. they survived symptoms of acute illness without being given fever suppressants, antibiotics or vaccines. It remains to be seen how future generations of adults will fare, since their childhoods have not been shaped by the same degree of experience with illness. Is there some connection between the suppression of infections and worldwide epidemic increases in weakness and functional disorders of the immune system, as expressed in many different allergies due to hypersensitivity of the surface organs (skin, lungs, intestines)?

Today, too, we can no longer speak convincingly of 'childhood illnesses', because both the possibility of immunisation and the increasing isolation of people in the industrialised world has produced a temporal shift in infectious illnesses once considered typical of childhood. The incidence of measles, and in some countries chickenpox, for example, is now greatest in adolescents and adults.

The following sections are intended to give a concrete overview of the symptoms, risks and complications of the main infectious diseases experienced in childhood and to alleviate unfounded anxieties about them. Which illnesses a child must come to grips with and how they do so are not matters of coincidence but part of the child's individual destiny. Hence we will attempt to describe

the acute symptoms of childhood illnesses in a way that enables parents to support their sick children with as much confidence as possible. For the same reason, we have added a chapter on the purpose and meaning of these symptoms (see Chapter 15).

Chapter 13 on preventing illness provides the basic information needed for making individualised, well-considered choices with regard to available immunisations.

7.1 Measles

A diagnosis of measles should always be confirmed by a doctor. Have your doctor examine your child at home if possible. If you cannot avoid moving your child, for example, if you have to take them to the hospital, make sure they remain lying down at all times.

The combined symptoms of measles have a considerable impact. Your child will likely feel exhausted and avoid light; their eyes may be reddened and slitted; their face may be bloated and red-speckled; their attempts to speak may produce only a deep, productive attack of coughing. However, significant improvement in symptoms should be evident around the third day after the beginning of the rash. The cough will persist for a week or longer. During the entire illness, it is important to ensure that your child gets the bed rest they so urgently need.

Causes
- Measles virus, Paramyxoviridae family

Symptoms
- There is an incubation period of 8–12 days to the beginning of the first stage, and 14 (occasionally 21) days to the appearance of the rash. There are usually 2 stages of measles:

First stage
- Moderate fever, runny nose, dry cough, throat ache, hoarseness, reddened eyes.
- Small white dots and 'spider webs' (Koplik's spots) appear on the mucous membranes lining the cheeks.

Second stage, 3–4 days later
- A second period of fever, usually higher, accompanied by the emergence of a rash.
- Fine red spots that appear first behind the ears and face, merging into a red rash covering large areas.
- Peaks around the second or third day of the rash appearing, then the fever subsides and the rash becomes paler.

- The cough may persist and diarrhoea is not uncommon.
- Sometimes the lymph nodes are affected.

Transmission
- Measles is highly contagious.
- The virus is spread by airborne droplets that are propelled many metres through coughing and sneezing.
- From day 9 after exposure until the fourth day after the rash appears, any children and adults who have been in contact with the patient can be affected.

Immunity
- Immunity is lifelong after a case of measles.
- An infant whose mother has had measles is fully protected by their antibodies for 4 months and partially protected for several more. If the mother has only been vaccinated, passive immunity is unreliable (see also page 272).
- Protection provided by vaccination: 93–95%.
- All children and adults who have been in contact with the patient during the contagious period must be considered infected. If they have been successfully immunised or have already had measles, this exposure will enhance their immunity as effectively as a booster shot.

Those whose vaccination was unsuccessful (about 5–7% of cases) may still come down with the illness unless they receive the vaccine again within 3 days.

• See page 272 for information on vaccination and adult measles.

Complications

In developed nations, complications are seldom a problem if children with measles are given extra rest and careful treatment, although caution is advised and experience in dealing with the illness is helpful. Severe pneumonia during measles is a rare but possible complication that can be fatal even in developed countries.

In the tropics and in countries that are less developed with regard to hygiene, standards of living and healthcare, the danger of measles is incomparably greater. In these countries, take local experience into account when deciding on prevention and treatment.

One empirical report from Africa, however, seems significant: mortality from measles was greatly reduced during one epidemic simply because no fever suppressants were administered. We do not recommend antipyretics (fever suppressants), but see Section 3.3 for recommendations for treating fever.

The following complications may occur:

• Temporarily lowered immunity for approximately 6 weeks after the illness; bacterial secondary infections develop in approximately 15 % of patients.
• Inflammation of the middle ear (otitis media – see page 33), sinusitis and pneumonia (see page 78) are not uncommon.
• Febrile seizures in 2% of cases.
• A series of seizures or a further period of rising fever accompanied by convulsions indicates acute measles-induced encephalitis: onset generally 3–9 days after the rash; incidence of 1:500 to 1:2,000 (see page 131).
• Subacute sclerosing panencephalitis (SSPE): onset approximately 5–10 years later; incidence 1–10 in 100,000 measles infections (see page 132).
• Flaring nostrils (see page 79) is a sign of pneumonia.

How you can help

• Always call a doctor.
• Ensure your child gets bed rest in a quiet, darkened room, with no background music or TV.
• Regulate the fever rather than make attempts to lower it (see page 56).
• Several times a day, note your child's pulse rate and respiratory rate, and record their temperature.
• Check for flaring nostrils (see

page 79), a sign of pneumonia.

- Have daily contact with your doctor, at home if at all possible.
- If you have to go to the doctor, call ahead before taking your child to avoid inadvertently exposing other children to the disease.
- Apply an onion pack for earache (see page 294).
- Use a chest compress (see page 298) for a cough. Apply thyme oil first, if the rash permits.
- Give your child plenty of time to recover.

Remedies

- **The homeopathic remedies and their dosages must be frequently adjusted by an experienced doctor.**
- Pulsatilla floribus 6X–12X glob. velati, 5 globules 3–6 times a day.
- Belladonna cum Mercurio glob. velati, 5 globules 4–8 times a day.
- For cough and pneumonia, Pneumodoron 1 and 2, alternating hourly: 5 drops in a little water (or, if necessary, the individual components: Phosphorus 8X, Aconitum 6X, Bryonia 4X, Tartarus stibiatus 4X).
- For earache, Apis/Levisticum I glob. velati, 5 globules 3–6 times a day.
- For eye irritation or conjunctivitis, Echinacea Quartz comp. eye drops, several times a day.
- For diarrhoea, Bolus alba comp.

powder, 1 teaspoon in ½ glass of water, 1 sip at a time.

Typical medications during 4–6 weeks of convalescence

- Meteoric iron glob. velati 5 globules 3 times a day, OR
- Rose iron/Graphite glob. velati 5 globules 3 times a day, OR
- Wala Prunuseisen glob. velati 5 globules 3 times a day, AND
- Additionally, as needed, Echinacea/Argentum glob. velati 5 globules 3 times a day

Convalescence

Your child's immune system will be weakened for several weeks after measles (depending on the severity of the illness). For this reason it is very important to allow adequate time for recovery. Consult your doctor about timing.

Acute encephalitis due to measles

Encephalitis is an inflammation of the brain. It is a possible complication of measles that affects between 1 in 500 and 1 in 2000 children, usually between the third and ninth day of the rash appearing. It is fatal in 10–20% of cases, and 20–30% of patients sustain lasting neurological damage. **If you suspect encephalitis, seek medical assistance immediately.**

Symptoms
- Headache
- Impairment of consciousness (up to and including coma, in extreme cases)
- Convulsions
- Neurological deficits (e.g. hemiplegia, a condition that affects movement on one side of the body)

Treatment
- A combination of the continuous supportive presence of a parent in the hospital, drug therapy for cerebral oedema and complementary medical treatment may positively influence the course of the illness.

SSPE (subacute sclerosing panencephalitis)
In rare cases, 5–10 years after contracting measles this severe degenerative form of encephalitis can develop if the patient has not succeeded in completely overcoming the measles viruses. Viral components that have not been adequately killed off remain in the body, especially in the brain, and then even relatively trivial triggers such as a measles vaccination at a later date can cause serious illness. Infants whose vaccinated mothers' placentas have not conveyed adequate maternal passive immunity are especially at risk.

There are about 4–11 cases per 100,000 cases of measles, although children under 5 show a higher incidence. The older the child is when contracting measles, the less likely they are to develop this complication. SSPE is often fatal and patients usually die 3–5 years after onset of the illness.

Symptoms
- Behavioural anomalies
- Intellectual changes
- Neurological deficits and disorders (convulsions)
- Loss of brain functions

7.2 German measles (rubella)

Causes
- Rubella virus, Togaviridae family.

Symptoms
- In 50% of cases there are no visible signs of illness.
- Possibly a rash of fine discrete red spots, beginning in the face and spreading to body and limbs, disappearing after 1–3 days.
- Possibly enlarged lymph nodes on both sides of the neck and behind the ears.
- Possibly a cold, conjunctivitis or a slight fever.
- Rash appears 2–3 weeks after exposure.

Transmission
- Transmission through airborne droplets.
- Contagious from 1 week before appearance of the rash to 1 week after the appearance of the rash.

Immunity
- Immunity is lifelong after a clear case of German measles.
- See page 270 for information on vaccination.

Complications
- Passing rheumatic diseases may develop in adolescents.
- Complications are very uncommon, although they do become somewhat more frequent with increasing age in cases of first-time infections: middle-ear infections, bronchitis, brain inflammation, heart muscle inflammation.
- Birth defects or stillbirths if infected during pregnancy, see below.

How you can help
- Bed rest as long as fever persists.
- Avoid physical exertion.

Remedies
- Echinacea/Argentum glob. velati, 5–10 globules in the morning and in the evening.
- For swelling of the lymph nodes, topical application of 10% Archangelica ointment.

German measles during pregnancy
Contracting rubella during the first 4 months of pregnancy may lead to miscarriage, preterm birth and congenital rubella syndrome (heart abnormalities, cataracts and inner-ear deafness) in the infant. The risk of damage declines later in the pregnancy, with the greatest risk existing between weeks 1 and 12 of gestation. After the fourth month of pregnancy, damage becomes infrequent.

7.3 Scarlet fever (scarlatina)

Causes
- Haemolytic strains of Streptococcus pyogenes (group A).

Symptoms
- There is an incubation period of 2–4 days.

Days 1 and 2
- Fever
- Sore throat
- Vomiting
- Difficulty swallowing
- Redness and swelling of the back edge of the gums
- Pustules on the uvula and tonsils

- White coating on the tongue that gives way to red bumps ('strawberry tongue').

Days 2 and 3
- Emergence of a dense, fine-grained rash (like red goose bumps), beginning in the arm-pits and groin and spreading upwards to the neck.
- Red cheeks but a pale triangle around the mouth and nose.
- Swelling of the cervical (neck) lymph nodes.

After 2–4 weeks
- Characteristic peeling of the skin on the palms and soles.

Transmission
- Through secretions, direct contact or contact with contam-inated objects or air, but usually only through close contact (sharing a room or dwelling).
- In acute untreated infection, patients are contagious for up to 3 weeks.
- With antibiotic treatment, con-tagiousness ends after 24 hours.
- Infants up to 3 years are rarely susceptible; the most susceptible are children between the ages of 6 and 12 years.

Quarantine
The patient should not attend public events until they have been treated with antibiotics for at least 48 hours and are symptom-free. Generally family members can attend public events 1 day after quarantining the patient or 1 day after treatment begins.

Immunity
- Because the immune system develops antibodies only against germ toxins (erythrogenic tox-ins), of which there are several in scarlet fever, and not against the germs themselves, recurrences of scarlet fever are possible.
- If the body already recognises the toxin, the only symptom of reinfection will be the sore throat.
- During epidemics, up to 25% of children may be symptom-free in spite of having the germs in their bodies; they are not consid-ered carriers of the disease.

Complications
Secondary infections are uncom-mon, and recent studies show that treatment with antibiotics does not prevent or decrease the risk. Even so, rheumatic fever is now much less common than in the early twentieth century, and especially in North America and Europe, nephritis also develops much less frequently. These shifts are attributed to socioeconomic and hygienic factors.

Under some circumstances, high fever that persists beyond day 4 may be a sign of *Kawasaki disease,* which has nothing to do with scarlet fever and must be treated differently. **Kawasaki disease, also known as mucocutaneous lymph node syndrome (MCLS), occurs most commonly in babies.** It is characterised by acute fever and its initial symptoms can look like scarlet fever or measles, but its cause has not yet been fully explained. It is accompanied by necrotising (tissue-destroying) vascular inflammation of the small and mid-sized arteries. This illness requires thorough examination and treatment, usually in a paediatric hospital. Approximately 1 in 10,000 children is affected by the disease.

Other complications of scarlet fever are rare, but if you are concerned and notice any of the following, check with your doctor.

Acute complications
- Inflammation of the middle ear (otitis media – see page 33).
- Toxicity with vomiting, diarrhoea, poor circulation, lethargy.
- Sepsis with meningitis (see page 27).

Secondary infections
- Rheumatic fever (see page 137), average onset 21 days after the streptococcus infection.

- Nephritis (see over page), average onset 10 days after the streptococcus infection.
- PANDAS (paediatric autoimmune neuropsychiatric disorders associated with streptococcal infections) neuropsychiatric symptoms such as tics, Tourette's syndrome, compulsive behaviours occur (very infrequently) weeks after the infection.

How you can help
- Bed rest.
- Light, low-fat diet.
- A long convalescent period: give your child at least 3 weeks before they resume their normal activities.
- The child should be examined again by a doctor if old symptoms persist (weakness, joint pains, oedema) or new ones (such as earaches) develop.

Treatment
Conventional treatment
Antibiotic treatment with penicillin for 10 days or cephalosporins for 5 days. The advantage of this treatment is that your child is no longer contagious after 24 hours. A systematic overview study of scarlet-fever sore throat, however, showed that antibiotic treatment was superior to placebo only for about 16 hours.

Anthroposophic treatment

In our paediatric practices, we meet many parents who want to avoid antibiotic treatment, especially when their children have already received penicillin several times for scarlet fever. In our experience, this is usually possible if good parent–doctor cooperation can be maintained.

Note, however, that avoiding antibiotics is not a safe option in situations where many people are living together (in group homes) or in developing countries. As a rule, family members are infected within a week, although whether or not they actually develop scarlet fever is another question. If a family member needs to avoid contagion, it is best for them to stay with relatives or friends for the duration. Isolating the patient, and preventative measures such as hand washing and wearing protective clothing in the sickroom, may not be effective in preventing the spread of the disease to other family members, although they are worth trying.

Any adult who deals professionally with children and develops a sore throat during a scarlet fever epidemic should be treated by a doctor. If requested, the entire family can be treated prophylactically with penicillin, but it may prevent infection for a short time only.

Although thorough examination by a doctor reveals no particular cause, children may still look pale and seem weak for a number of weeks after even mild cases of scarlet fever, because the disease is accompanied by strong breakdown processes that may affect or even damage organs. For this reason, we recommend that children who have had scarlet fever, even if treated with antibiotics, be allowed a long convalescent period: at least 3 weeks before resuming their normal activities.

Remedies

- Apis/Belladonna cum Mercurio glob. velati, 5 globules 6–8 times a day.
- Cinnabar comp., 1 pea-sized portion of powder 6–8 times a day, OR
- Echinacea/Argentum glob. velati, 5 globules in the morning and at midday for 4–6 weeks.
- Gargling with Bolus Eucalypti comp. or Wala Echinacea Mouth and Throat Spray, several times a day.

Nephritis/post-streptococcal glomerulonephritis (PSGN)

Nephritis affects the kidneys and means that the body cannot make as much urine as usual. In the great majority of cases, this type of kidney inflammation can be completely cured.

Symptoms

- Blood in the urine 10 days to 5 weeks after the streptococcal infections.
- Foamy, frothy or bubbly-looking urine may be a sign of increased protein elimination 10 days to 5 weeks after the streptococcal infection.
- Sometimes accompanied by high blood pressure and reduced urination.
- Swelling (oedema) of the eyelids and/or ankles may occur.
- In addition, children may appear generally unwell, with pallor, loss of appetite, headaches and vomiting.
- As a rule, symptoms persist for 1–2 weeks, but blood and protein may be present in the urine for up to 18 months.

Treatment

- Antibiotics
- Cortisone in severe cases
- Bed rest and avoiding exertion
- Treatment for high blood pressure, if needed

Remedies

- Equisetum cum Sulfure tostum 6X, 1 pea-sized portion of powder 3–6 times a day.
- Cardiodoron, 5 drops 3–6 times a day.
- Kidney rubs with 0.4% Cuprum metallicum praep. ointment, in the evenings.

Rheumatic fever

This illness attacks primarily the joints and the heart.

Symptoms

- Pallor, fatigue, loss of appetite, abdominal pain and fever develop approximately 2–6 weeks after a streptococcal infection.
- Joint inflammation (redness, swelling and heat), generally around the large joints but possibly moving into other joints. Symptoms disappear within 24 hours after beginning anti-inflammatory treatment.
- Carditis (inflammation of the heart) is the most dangerous complication. All layers of the cardiac wall can be affected. In the worst cases, myocardial insufficiency develops, along with permanent damage to the heart valves, which then result in cardiac abnormalities.

Treatment

Treatment must always be administered in a hospital and generally involves antibiotics. If the heart is affected, acetylsalicylic acid (aspirin) and cortisone may also be used.

7.4 Roseola (3-day fever, exanthema subitum)

Roseola is a common viral infection that **causes a fever and a spotty rash. It is common among infants and children.**

Causes
• Humanes herpes type-6 viruses (HHV-6).

Symptoms
• High fever (up to 40°C/104°F), usually for 3 days, sometimes up to 5 days.
• After the fever falls, a rash of fine red spots on the trunk and nape of the neck, sometimes spreading to face and limbs.
• Incubation period is 5–15 days.

Transmission
• The disease is usually transmitted by infectious saliva (the parents are probably the primary source of infection) but possibly also by airborne droplets.
• It is most common in the first year of life; by age 2 almost all children have experienced this infection.

Immunity
• Lifelong

Complications
Usually appearing in the first few days:
• Gastrointestinal infection
• Cough
• Swelling of the cervical lymph nodes
• Swelling of the eyelids
• Fever with a bulging fontanelle, sometimes mimicking meningitis (see also page 27)
• Febrile seizures, harmless in most cases

How you can help
• See Fever, page 54.
• If symptoms of meningitis show (see page 27), take your child to a doctor immediately or call emergency services.

Remedies
• As for Fever, see page 54.
• Apis/Belladonna glob. velati, 5 globules 3–6 times a day.
• Echinacea/Argentum glob. velati, 5 globules, morning and afternoon, for 2 weeks.

7.5 Slapped cheek syndrome/fifth disease (erythema infectiosum)

Slapped cheek syndrome gets its name from a characteristic rash on both cheeks, although in many cases the disease is symptomless. It is common in children and should clear up by itself within 3 weeks.

Cause
- Parvovirus B19

Symptoms
- In most cases it is symptomless.
- Possibly 2–3 days of flu-like respiratory symptoms without rash.
- The typical rash develops only in 15–20% of patients, mainly children. It begins as large red spots on the cheeks that merge in a butterfly-like shape. As in scarlet fever, there is often a pale triangle around the mouth and nose. With time the rash spreads to the trunk and limbs, where it manifests as an itchy maculopapular rash in a lacy pattern with pale centres.
- The rash can recur anywhere from 1–7 weeks after it disappears.
- The incubation period is 4–14 days.

Transmission
- Transmitted by airborne droplets and on the hands of infected individuals.
- Most contagious during the first 4–10 days; once the rash appears, your child is generally no longer contagious.

Immunity
- After contracting the disease once, immunity is usually life-long; infection rates vary considerably in different parts of the world.

Complications
- Transitory joint pain and inflammation may appear, primarily in girls and young women.
- Other complications are very uncommon.
- If a pregnant woman is infected, there is not usually a problem. The risk of the foetus contracting the disease ranges from 5–10%, or up to 15% if the infection occurs between weeks 13 and 20 of gestation. However, in rare cases it can lead to the foetus becoming severely anaemic or even to miscarriage.

How you can help
- Ensure that your child avoids exertion, especially when joint symptoms are present.
- Stannum metallicum 0.4% ointment wraps on the painful joints.

Remedies
- Echinacea/Argentum glob. velati, 5 globules in the morning and in the evening.
- Rhus toxicodendron comp. glob. velati, 5 globules 3–6 times a day for joint symptoms.

- Blood transfusions are attempted when the infection induces anaemia in an embryo.

7.6 Chickenpox (varicella)

This disease is harmless, but it is dreaded in hospitals because it can be transmitted through air-conditioning systems and endangers patients with weakened immunity. Do not visit hospitals if chickenpox is suspected.

Cause
- Varicella zoster virus

Symptoms
- Itching, irregularly distributed spots appear, usually on the body and face at first, rapidly developing into fluid-filled blisters that form scabs before healing.
- The blisters also appear on the limbs, scalp and the palms of hands, on the genitals and in the mouth.
- Mild, brief fever is possible.
- Occasionally there is a 'silent' infection without symptoms or only a few, hardly noticeable blisters.
- The incubation period is 14–16 days.

Transmission
- Highly contagious.
- Transmission is through airborne droplets. Casual exposure, even through an open door or window, is sufficient.
- The contagious period begins 1–2 days before symptoms appear and ends when the last blisters have dried up; it's possible, for those with a weak immune system, that the contagious period lasts until the final crust has fallen off.

Immunity
- Lifelong immunity through a wild virus (the naturally occurring, non-mutated form of a virus).
- Infants are immune for the first few months of life if their mothers have had chickenpox.
- For vaccination advice, see page 269.
- The virus may be reactivated and reappear later in life in the form of *shingles (herpes zoster)* when immunity is low, as the virus remains in the nerve ganglia. The shingles rash of small raised dots appears only in a band on the skin that corresponds to the location of a cutaneous nerve most commonly on the torso, but all other parts of the body are also possible. The rash is often

painful and persistent high fever may also occur. When another member of the family has herpes zoster, children are sometimes infected and contract chickenpox.

Complications

- Complications are infrequent.
- Bacterial infections, e.g. abscesses.
- Symptoms are more severe in individuals predisposed to neurodermatitis.
- Pneumonia is uncommon in children, but more frequent in adults.
- Complications that affect the nervous system are very uncommon.
- The disease is much more serious in immunocompromised individuals: pneumonia and encephalitis are possible. Newborns whose mothers contract chickenpox anywhere from 5 days before delivery until 2 days after the birth require treatment with antivirals and immunoglobulins.
- If a pregnant woman contracts chickenpox for the first time in approximately weeks 8–24 of gestation, congenital varicella syndrome with severe abnormalities is possible in the foetus, although very uncommon.

How you can help

- Apply a soothing powder, such as Weleda Wecesin, to the itching areas of skin.
- For *intact blisters*, apply a burns gel like Combudoron.
- To *relieve severe itching*, have a lukewarm bath or wash with marigold (calendula) flower tea.
- For a *rash in the genital area*, have a bath containing chamomile tea.
- For a *rash in the mouth*, use Weleda mouthwash.
- For *concurrent neurodermatitis*, use Imlan pur or Argan-clay lotion (Pekur).
- For *bacterial secondary infections*, dab the affected areas with thyme tea and add it to bath water.

Remedies

- Echinacea/Argentum glob. velati, 5 globules in the morning and evening for 2–3 weeks.

After chickenpox

- Infected blisters may leave small scars as they heal, but these usually disappear with time. Rosatum Heilsalbe is good for healing scars.

7.7 Mouth ulcers (herpes simplex stomatitis)

Herpes simplex stomatitis involves repeated episodes of mouth ulcers: flat, greyish, painful craters up to the size of lentils that develop in the mucous membranes of the mouth. It usually affects young children between the ages of 10 months and 3 years.

Single mouth ulcers that persist for a few days or weeks and are not contagious have nothing in common with herpes simplex stomatitis, except the pain they cause.

Cause
• Herpes simplex virus type 1

Symptoms
• Pronounced bad breath.
• Usually accompanied by high fever.
• Difficulty swallowing, which can lead to not taking in food or (in severe cases) fluids.
• Increased salivation.
• Many painful blisters and ulcers on the tongue, inside the cheeks, on the gums, lips and around the mouth.
• Incubation period is 3–7 days.

Transmission
• Transmission occurs through bodily contact or airborne droplets e.g. using same dishes or cutlery.

Immunity
• Partial immunity only: lifelong recurrences of cold sores (fever blisters) are possible. See Fever blisters (cold sores, herpes simplex), page 106.

Complications
• Very rarely, meningitis or pneumonia in newborn babies or people with reduced immunity.
• In children with neurodermatitis, the disease may be serious and large areas of skin can be affected.

How you can help
• **Ensure there can be no contact with newborn babies.**
• Rinsing with mouth balsam (Wala Mundbalsam gel) relieves symptoms as it is slightly anaesthetising and anti-inflammatory. Dilute with same amount of water. If it still has a burning senation, dilute more.
• Pure honey may also help.
• Children with herpes simplex stomatitis often refuse to eat because swallowing is painful, but weight lost is rapidly regained.
• Ensure your child drinks enough

to prevent dehydration. Hospi-talisation is required in severe cases of dehydration.

Remedies

- Cinnabar comp., 1 pinch 4–6 times a day.
- Apis/Belladonna cum Mercurio, 5 globules 4–6 times a day.
- Echinacea/Argentum glob. velati, 5 globules, morning and after-noon, for 4 weeks.

7.8 Mumps (epidemic parotitis)

Mumps has become relatively rare in recent years, but when it does appear, symptoms and their severity vary considerably. The meninges can be affected and produce symptoms of viral meningitis (see page 27). This condition may go unrecognised, but fortunately it is almost always harmless in children. It is often possible to avoid hospitalisation, and lumbar puncture is almost never necessary. Antibiotic treat-ment is useless, since mumps is a viral infection.

Cause

- Mumps virus (paramyxoviridae family)

Symptoms

- In 30–40% of cases there are no symptoms.
- Fever and painful swelling of the parotid glands (salivary glands located below each ear), either on both sides or on one side only.
- Pain when chewing, reddened excretory ducts of salivary glands, protruding ear lobes.
- Mild abdominal pain, nausea and vomiting may occur.
- Duration of swelling is 3–7 days.
- Incubation period is 16–18 days.

Transmission

- Transmission by airborne drop-lets.
- The contagious period extends from 3 days before the appear-ance of symptoms to 9 days after.
- Maternal passive immunity dur-ing the first 6 months.

Immunity

- Generally lifelong after illness, but less reliable if only through vaccination. For vaccination see page 270.

Complications

- Complications may appear as late as 2 weeks after the begin-ning of the illness.
- *Viral meningitis* may appear 4–5 days after swelling and lasts 7–10 days. It is the most common complication in children, but

it is a condition without consequences and is not even noticed in 70% of cases.

- *Encephalitis* is a rare complication (under 1%), appearing 4–5 days after swelling. Symptoms: neurological deficit, vomiting, drowsiness or lethargy (see page 131).
- *Inflammation of the testes* is very rare with children, though will occur in 20–30% of cases of mumps in adult men. It appears 4–8 days after mumps and lasts 1–2 weeks. In 13% of cases, fertility may be affected. However, becoming sterile as a result of mumps is extremely rare, even if both testes are affected.
- Comparable inflammation of the ovaries is possible in females but is generally harmless.
- Inflammation of the pancreas in about 4% of cases.
- Infrequently, mumps causes hearing loss (the incidence is said to be 1 in every 10–15,000 cases).
- Data on the frequency of such complications needs to be evaluated critically, since they are influenced by geographical, cultural and individual constitutional factors and may also reflect epidemics or inadequate treatment.

How you can help
- Ensure your child rests.
- Apply archangelica ointment or warm compresses made with calendula (marigold) oil (see page 302) to the cheeks (not the head).
- For abdominal pain, apply warm, moist compresses made with chamomile or yarrow tea.
- Ensure your child has a fat-free diet.
- Do not attempt to reduce the fever, even if it is high, except on the advice of your doctor. Fever may lessen the possibility of complications by reducing viral activity.

Remedies
- Archangelica comp. glob. velati, 5 globules 4 times daily.
- Apis/Belladonna glob. velati, 5 globules 4 times daily.
- Argentum metallicum praep. 12X 1 pinch 3 times a day, or Echinacea/Argentum glob. velati, 5 globules, morning and afternoon.
- If pancreas is affected: Cichorium/Pancreas comp. glob. velati, 5 globules, 4–6 times daily.
- Mercurius vivus nat. 6X 1 tablet 3 times a day.

7.9 Whooping cough (pertussis)

Cause
- Bordetella pertussis bacterium

Symptoms
There are three stages:

1. Catarrhal stage
- Runny nose
- Elevated temperature
- Unusual cough
- Conjunctivitis
- Duration: 1–2 weeks

2. Acute stage
- Temperature usually returns to normal.
- Increasing attacks of coughing, especially at night (intense coughing, face can turn red and then blue, loud gulping noises when breathing in, retching up thick phlegm, often ends in vomiting).
- Typically there are periods in which there are no symptoms.
- Duration: 4–6 weeks

3. Convalescent stage
- Coughing fits become less frequent and decline
- Duration: 2–4 weeks

Incubation period
- 7–14 days

Transmission
- Airborne droplets
- Susceptibility is highest during the first (catarrhal) stage, with 70–80% of contacts developing whooping cough.

Immunity
- Recurrences are possible
- **Infants are not protected by maternal antibodies**
- For vaccination, see page 266

Complications
- Pneumonia (see page 78)
- Inflammation of the middle ear (otitis media – see page 33)
- Convulsions in 2–4% of cases
- Fatal respiratory failure – very rarely in infants in the first 3 months of life

How you can help
- Avoid contact with infants.
- Give your child plenty to drink.
- Do not give chemical sedatives or cough suppressants, because these drugs reduce the frequency and intensity of coughing. As a result, phlegm is more likely to remain in the lungs, where it can contribute to the development of pneumonia and oxygen deficiency in the brain.
- Apply chest compresses with lavender or thyme oil (see page 301).

- Apply a thin layer of Cuprum metallicum praep. 0.1% ointment between the shoulder blades.

How to help during an attack of coughing

- When children have an attack of coughing, do not clap them on the back, pull them out of bed or show other signs of excitement. This does nothing to shorten the attack and will only make the situation worse for an already upset child.
- To help inhalation, support the forehead lightly and rub your child's back while saying soothing words, such as 'Go ahead, cough it all up. Good. Now take a breath and cough again,' to let your child know that everything is as it should be and there is no need to panic. Your calm presence is often the only help your child needs.
- Little children who lie on their stomachs may raise themselves up on their arms until the coughing fit is over and then lie down again.
- Ideally, one parent should sleep on an extra bed in the child's room, so that someone is available to clean up vomit if needed and replace the protective covering on the child's bed.

Prevention

In babies less than 3 months old, whooping cough is dangerous, because young infants have difficulty coughing effectively. Brain complications are possible. All parents must know how to prevent infection in their newborn or young infant:

- Adults or children who are coughing or fighting infections should avoid the infant's room.
- If the parents themselves are affected, they should wear masks.
- Only children who are quite definitely healthy should be allowed into the newborn's room.

Whooping cough in a kindergarten or neighbourhood is a risk to infant siblings of older children who have not had the disease, and their parents should be alerted if a case occurs. Your doctor can take necessary measures if you suspect your infant has been infected. Administering a narrow-spectrum antibiotic can prevent the infection from developing in newly infected infants.

If your young infant is infected

Susceptibility to whooping cough is almost 100% in newborns, even among breastfed babies. **If you suspect that your infant has been exposed, monitor them constantly and consult your doctor.**

Your baby should be hospitalised as soon as symptoms appear, and the prognosis is generally better if a parent is admitted along with the child.

Infants between the ages of 3 and 6 months can also become seriously ill with whooping cough, but in most cases they are able to cough more effectively than very young babies. Depending on the circumstances and the experience of parents and doctor, antibiotic treatment may still be advisable.

In children older than 1 year, complications are rare except in situations of neglect and antibiotic treatment is no longer needed. We have often been able to dispense with it in otherwise healthy children over the age of 3 months.

Whooping cough is significantly more dangerous in children who have rickets or whose diet is low in calcium. For this reason, we always recommend examination by a doctor when the acute stage of whooping cough becomes evident in a child less than 1 year old.

After whooping cough

Bouts of coughing can recur months later, whenever the child contracts a new infection, even though they are no longer contagious. It has long been known that whooping cough rarely leads to asthma or allergies and has nothing to do with recent increases in these diseases.

Treatment

- Antibiotics can be considered if you would prefer your child not to experience the normal course of the illness, or to avoid complications in infants and children with severe asthma. However, note that antibiotic treatment should be started in the catarrhal stage, since later use of antibiotics will not influence the progression of the disease.
- Very young babies may initially need to be hospitalised for monitoring and antibiotic therapy. Treatment may then be continued at home as long as a baby monitor is used.
- Preventative antibiotics may be recommended for infants and children with pre-existing cardiac and respiratory conditions who have been in close contact with infected individuals.

Anthroposophic therapy

- Weleda Pertudoron 1 and 2 in alternation, 5 drops up to once every hour.
- Your doctor may also prescribe single homeopathic remedies such as Drosera 6X, Ipecacuanha 4X, and/or Tabacum Cupro cultum Rh 3X.

7.10 Diphtheria

In the early nineteenth century, diphtheria was considered one of the most dangerous childhood diseases and mortality rates were high. Nowadays, the disease is very uncommon in affluent countries. However, diphtheria still exists in tropical Africa, the Indian subcontinent and Southeast Asia where there is inadequate vaccination.

Diphtheria is remarkable among serious contagious diseases for the extent to which a full-blown case suppresses the patient's endogenous forces. Although the patient does not develop a high fever, they look pale and their pulse is rapid and weak, and their blood pressure tends to be low. The disease is characterised by internal toxemia (blood poisoning) that affects the circulatory and nervous systems in particular.

Cause

Corynebacterium diphtheriae (Klebs-Löffler bacillus)

Symptoms

A variety of different manifestations are possible:

- *Diphtheria of the tonsils and throat:* fever, difficulty swallowing, lethargy, painfully swollen cervical lymph nodes, reddened tonsils with greyish-white coating that extends to the gums and is difficult to remove, sweetish putrid mouth odour.
- *Diphtheria of the nose:* most common in infants; bloody/watery nasal discharge that forms crusts.
- *Diphtheria of the larynx:* hoarseness, barking cough, wheezing inhalation, respiratory distress, risk of suffocation.
- *Diphtheria of the skin:* this is uncommon, but may occur on all mucous membranes and sensitive areas of skin such as the navel or wounds, where greasy coatings develop.
- Incubation period is 2–5 days.

Susceptibility and transmission

- Bacteria are spread through airborne droplets.
- Close contact with an infected person.
- Animals may also transmit the bacteria.
- Contagious as long as the pathogen can be found in secretions and wounds, generally for a period of 2 weeks without treatment though seldom longer than 4 weeks, and approximately 2–4 days with antibiotic treatment.

Immunity

- Recurrences are possible (see Vaccinations, page 265).

Complications

- Complications are caused by the bacterial toxin and may show after the second week of illness.
- Heart and circulatory failure due to bacterial blood poisoning, possibly fatal.
- Temporary paralysis of the soft palate or eye muscles due to inflammation of nerves.
- Kidney failure, encephalitis or endocarditis are possible but rare.

How you can help

- **Hospitalisation is required. Early treatment of suspected diphtheria is essential.**

Treatment

- Antitoxins and antibiotics (penicillin).
- *For throat diphtheria:* a pinch of Cinnabar comp. 6–8 times daily.
- *For larynx diphtheria:* Bryonia/ Spongia comp. 5–10 drops in water 6–8 times daily.
- Echinacea/Argentum glob. velati, 5 globules, morning and afternoon, for 4 weeks.
- As an additional measure during convalescence, restoration of the intestinal flora with probiotics.

7.11 Glandular fever (infectious mononucleosis, Epstein-Barr virus)

Cause

- Epstein-Barr virus (herpes family)

Symptoms

Glandular fever is a diagnostic chameleon, capable of presenting a great variety of symptoms and different progressions, so it is always a possibility to be considered in ambiguous cases. Possible symptoms include:

- High fever
- Pronounced swelling of the lymph nodes
- Tonsillitis, usually with extensive white coatings that do not extend to the palate
- Spleen and liver enlargement, with a mild rash and jaundice
- In infants and toddlers, the infection may manifest as a respiratory infection
- Incubation period is 10–50 days

Transmission

- Through infected saliva, hence the common name 'kissing disease'.
- The disease can still be transmitted through intimate contact for several months after initial symptoms appear.

Immunity

- Usually lasting, except in individuals with weakened immune systems (i.e. after chemotherapy there may be relapse or chronic recurrences).
- **Individuals who have had glandular fever should avoid immunisations for the next 4 months until the immune system is fully functional again.**

Complications

Complications are unusual in children, but may include the following:

- Disorders of the central nervous system, such as Guillain-Barré syndrome, encephalitis (see page 131)
- Reduced function of blood cell formation, such as a reduction in platelets and red blood cells
- Myocarditis (heart muscle inflammation)
- Nephritis (see page 136)
- Skin rash (e.g. in a patient wrongly treated with penicillin)
- Rupture of the spleen

How you can help

- Ensure your child has bed rest in the acute phase.
- Let your child have at least 4 weeks without sports or physical exertion to avoid rupture of the spleen and to aid speedy recovery.

Remedies

- Archangelica ointment may be used externally for easing the swelling of the lymph nodes.
- Stannum metallicum 0.4% liver compress at night, if required.
- Gargling, e.g. with Bolus Eucalypti comp., several times a day.
- Mercurius vivus nat. 6X,1 tablet 3–4 times a day.

7.12 Infectious hepatitis, type A

Hepatitis A is the most common but least dangerous type of liver infection in children.

Cause

- Hepatitis, type A virus

Symptoms

- Children often don't show any symptoms of Hepatitis A, or only very slight ones.
- *Early stage:* tiredness, lack of appetite, nausea or vomiting, abdominal pain, possibly diarrhoea and fever.
- *Course of the illness:* possibly signs of bile congestion (itching, dark brown urine, pale stools); liver and sometimes the spleen are enlarged. This phase can last from a few days to several weeks.
- *Recovery period:* symptoms lessen during this period, which

can last from 2–4 weeks.
- Incubation period can be 15–50 days, but generally 25–30 days.

Transmission
- Transmission is 'fecal-oral' and generally occurs through close personal contact, or unclean food, water and utensils.
- When travelling to high-risk countries, follow this common-sense rule: 'Peel it, cook it or leave it.'
- Susceptibility is 1 or 2 weeks before symptoms appear to 1 week afterwards.

Immunity
- Lifelong immunity after completed infection
- For vaccination, see page 276

Complications
- In about 10% of cases the illness can take several months to develop, though recovery is without further complications.
- In 0.01–0.1% (rising with age), there may be complications leading to liver failure.

How you can help
- Ensure your child gets bed rest.
- Warm yarrow tea compresses applied to the liver area (see page 304), or Stannum metallicum 0.4% ointment.
- An easily digestible diet.

Remedies
- Fragaria/vitis comp. (Hepata-doron) tablets, 1–3 tablets every evening.
- Taraxacum planta tota, 5 drops 3–4 times daily, or Taraxacum Stanno cultum Rh 3X, 5 drops 3–4 times daily before meals.

7.13 Infectious hepatitis, type B

Hepatitis B is a liver infection spread through blood and bodily fluids. In contrast to hepatitis A, hepatitis B is potentially harmful to children in the long-term. If untreated, the infection can last for years and eventually cause liver damage. **Seek medical advice if you suspect your child has hepatitis B.**

Cause
- Hepatitis, type B virus

Symptoms
In over 50% of cases of hepatitis B in infants and toddlers, symptoms are absent or only very slight. However, they may include:
- *Early stages of the illness:* fever, vomiting or diarrhoea, lasting 2–3 weeks.
- *Course of the illness:* enlargement of liver and spleen, jaundice, itching, dark brown urine, pale stools.

151

- Incubation period is from 45–180 days, but on average 60–120 days.

Transmission

Transmission is through infected body fluids (blood, semen, saliva, rarely breast milk). Newborns can pick up hepatitis B from their mothers and in countries where the infection is common, the infection is easily spread from child to child within families.

Immunity

- Lifelong immunity after completed infection.
- For vaccination, see page 277.

Complications

- Acute hepatitis B becomes serious in approximately 1% of cases.
- Whether the disease becomes chronic depends on the patient's age at first infection: approximately 95% of newborns, 25–40% of toddlers and 1–5% of school-age children and adults.
- Cirrhosis of the liver.
- Cancer of the liver.

How you can help

- Always seek medical advice
- See Hepatitis A (page 150)

Treatment

- Anthroposophic medicines as for Hepatitis A.

- Conventional treatment: Interferon therapy may be used to inhibit replication of the virus.

Prevention

- After birth, active and passive immunisation for newborns with hepatitis B positive mothers.
- Medical personnel should be immunised or wear gloves.
- For vaccination see page 277.

7.14 Lyme disease (borreliosis)

Lyme disease is a bacterial infection usually spread to humans by infected ticks. The earlier it is treated the better.

When removing a tick from your child's skin, some of its biting apparatus may remain behind in the skin. As a rule, this foreign body is expelled spontaneously, but a strong local reaction or inflammation is possible. **Lyme disease can have serious consequences: always seek medical advice**.

Cause

- Borrelia burgdorferi bacterium

Symptoms

Symptoms and progression of Lyme disease vary greatly but most frequently appear on the skin and in the nervous system, joints and heart. Occasionally an infection will be completely asymptomatic. Possible symptoms include:

- Flu-like symptoms are possible at various stages.
- *A bull's eye rash* (Erythema migrans) appears in only about 50% of infections. Days to weeks after the tick bite, a clearly delineated, painless red spot appears and then spreads outwards, becoming pale in the centre.
- Lymphocytoma cutis sometimes develops simultaneously as a bluish-red swelling. In children, it is most common on the ears.
- Skin symptoms may be accompanied by fever, headache, muscle pain, conjunctivitis or swelling of the lymph nodes.

Early spreading of the infection to different organs

- *Neuroborreliosis* with meningitis or inflammation of individual nerves in the head. In children, borreliosis is the most common cause of facial nerve paralysis, which eventually resolves completely.
- More common in adults is extremely painful radiculitis (inflammation of nerve roots in the spinal cord).
- Myocarditis (heart muscle inflammation) may also occur.

Late or chronic-phase manifestations, which persist beyond 6 months

- Chronic joint inflammation, especially of the knee joint.
- Chronic skin damage, especially reddish-blue discolouration and extreme thinning of the skin on the legs.
- Chronic neurological disorders, pain and states of exhaustion.

Incubation period

- Early manifestation can be weeks to months; late manifestations can be months to years.

Transmission

- Transmitted by bites from ticks infected with the bacterium Borrelia burgdorferi.
- Risk of infection increases the longer the tick is attached.
- Not contagious; no human-to-human transmission.
- Immunity.
- No lifelong immunity: recurrence always possible.
- There is currently no vaccination.

Complications

- Generally early recognition and treatment of tick bites means there are no complications.
- It is more difficult to treat Lyme disease at the late stage, when concomitant illnesses and complications can arise.

How you can help

- If you go for a walk in fields, woodland or a tick-infested area, wear clothing to cover most of your skin.
- As soon as you return from your walk, check yourself and your children for ticks from head to toe. If it is not possible to do so immediately, at least ensure you do so before the end of the day.
- Anti-tick repellants can be used, but lose their effectiveness after about 2 hours. If there are no allergies, try etheric oils, such as lavender, thyme, cypress, cedar, lemon, lemongrass or neem extract.
- If you find a tick, remove it with special tweezers. Apply light pressure to the skin, so the tweezers can grasp the tick's head. Do not crush the tick's body. Pull the tick out without twisting.
- If no tools are available, use a cotton thread rather than delay. Tie a loop around the tick's mouthparts as close to the skin as possible and then pull upwards without twisting.
- Disinfect the bite, the tools and your hand.

- If small hooks of the tick's biting apparatus remain embedded in the skin, they will be expelled naturally after a tiny inflammatory reaction.
- With any signs of illness, ensure rest.

Treatment

- Antibiotics to treat circular rash, neuroborreliosis, arthritis and inflammation of the heart muscle.

Remedies

- *After tick bite and with neuroborreliosis:* Argentum/quartz glob. velati, 5 globules, morning and afternoon.
- *To strengthen the immune system:* Echinacea/Argentum glob. velati, 5 globules, morning and afternoon.
- *With flu-like symptoms:* Levico comp. glob. velati, 5 globules, 3 times daily.
- *With headaches and aching limbs:* Gelsemium comp. glob. velati, 5 globules, 3 times daily.
- Restoration of intestinal flora with probiotics after antibiotic treatment.

8. Diabetes

8.1 Type 1 diabetes

When we talk about juvenile diabetes, what we usually mean is insulin-dependent Type 1 diabetes, which requires lifelong administration of insulin. When we eat and drink, our bodies process the food and break it down into glucose. Insulin allows the glucose to enter the cells of our bodies. Usually the pancreas produces insulin; however, with diabetes the pancreas cannot produce insulin, which means blood glucose levels become too high.

Children who are diagnosed with Type 1 diabetes learn to shoulder responsibility at a very young age. They must assess their activity levels and consider what they eat more carefully. Indeed, the whole family, through dealing with insulin injections, blood-sugar monitoring and accurate assessment of the child's metabolic situation, learns to substitute deliberate thought and action for the cellular function (insulin production) that has been destroyed by an autoimmune process in the pancreas.

We can get a glimpse of the meaning and impact of this illness in the child's individual destiny, in their family and in larger social contexts (for example, kindergarten, school, vacations and later higher education and a career) when we experience the special abilities acquired through living with diabetes, which can include: more mature levels of self-perception, self-management and self-assurance; confidence in choosing friends; greater family cohesiveness; and exceptional reliability, planning and forethought.

Causes of Type 1 diabetes

Onset of Type 1 diabetes peaks in childhood. In recent decades, Type 1 diabetes has increased in our society, and children are being affected more frequently. It is difficult to catch early because by the time symptoms appear, the self-destructive inflammatory process that attacks the insulin-producing islet cells in the pancreas is already up to 90% complete.

According to the present state of our knowledge, the causes of this process and thus of the diabetic condition are very complex. Having parents or siblings with Type 1 diabetes increases a child's chances of contracting the disease at some point in life by 5–10%. We also believe that some of the factors involved are related to our modern lifestyle. Type 1 diabetes can be successfully managed, but there is not yet a cure.

Warning signs

- Your child is drinking significantly more than usual
- Increased trips to the toilet at night
- Exhaustion, weakness
- Poor concentration
- Weight loss, even though your child's food intake remains consistent

Initial treatment and diabetes education

If diagnosed with Type 1 diabetes, your child will usually be hospitalised for anywhere from 8–14 days while you and your family learn how to manage daily life with the new diagnosis. The presence of both parents is highly desirable in terms of the future course of the disease.

There is a great deal of new information available about insulin, metabolism, nutrition, physical activity and how they all relate to blood sugar balance. Your family will also learn necessary practical techniques: how to monitor blood sugar, administer insulin and calculate the number of units needed, and recognise and treat low and high blood sugar.

Frequent monitoring is needed in order to calculate insulin doses correctly, especially for little children who cannot yet say when they aren't feeling well.

In the course of the first weeks and months, your family will become used to the new daily routine, and become more relaxed in dealing with diabetes. Grandparents and siblings can also get involved.

Early on in particular, families often hear a lot of alarming information or misinformation, such as that low blood sugar is life-threatening, a diabetic child can never eat sugar again, diabetes is due to stress or poor eating habits etc. The best course of action is to educate yourselves and others around you. In schools and kindergartens, it is vital to apprise all the teachers and caregivers of your child's diabetes, so that everyone knows what to do, especially in instances of low blood sugar or when readings are not what they should be. Diabetes will be an inescapable part your child's daily life from now on and will require due consideration from everyone involved in their care.

The reliable support of a juvenile diabetes treatment team is important from the very beginning. For children and teens under age 16, treatment should be overseen by a juvenile diabetologist who has received specialised training in dealing with this age group. They are experienced in supporting young diabetics to develop autonomy with regard to their illness and encourage them to deal self-confidently and independently with it at home and in kindergarten or school.

Out-patient follow-up appointments should be scheduled approximately every 2 months to discuss not only the treatment and its implementation, but also everyday experiences with it and what can be learned from them.

Living a 'normal' and fulfilling life

It is respectful to bear in mind that diabetic children have an additional full-time job of consciously adapting their metabolism to the changing circumstances of their life, reflecting on their activity level and body perceptions and adjusting their actions accordingly. Your child will appreciate people acknowledging and appreciating this extra 'work': for example, if their teachers ask how they are and how it's going with the diabetes. That being said, remember that your child can have a normal and fulfilling life, and they will benefit from being treated as such.

Your child's life situation should not be altered to accommodate treatment; rather, treatment should be adapted to the circumstances of real life. The issue is not how to make your child compatible with living with diabetes, but rather finding a child-appropriate way of dealing with the disease. Encourage your child to approach their diabetes with confidence and model that behaviour yourself. To conceal dealing with insulin, whether by administering it under the desk or in the bathroom, does not help but simply makes daily life more difficult.

Artistic therapies and curative eurythmy can help with self-confidence. Reliable professional support can also help prevent fears of 'bad' blood sugar levels, hypoglycaemic incidents and other consequences of the disease as well as diabetes-related intra-familial conflicts or feelings of guilt from dominating the daily treatment routine. Instead, what is learned through coming to grips with diabetes can increasingly become a 'competency bank' that both your child and your family will be able to draw on for a lifetime.

Insulin therapy

Insulin therapy is usually administered in concentrated form using insulin 'pens', which involves multiple injections per day. This type of therapy makes it possible for children to continue to eat age-appropriately and without dietary restrictions due to the illness. Type 1 diabetes does not require a special diet.

An insulin pump that dispenses insulin constantly, as opposed to multiple larger injections, closely imitates the physiological rhythm of the metabolism and is recommended for babies and toddlers. In healthy individuals, the islet cells in the pancreas make insulin available according to a characteristic day/night rhythm. The pump dispenses an individually calibrate dose of insulin via a thin tube inserted into subcutaneous fatty tissue (e.g. in the abdomen). And at each meal, the appropriate amount of insulin calculated on the basis of food and beverages consumed can be dispensed via the skin into the fatty tissue and from there into the blood, which makes many aspects of daily life less complicated.

Low or high blood sugar?

Monitoring blood sugar levels is essential with diabetes. Low blood sugar (hypoglycaemia) or high blood sugar (hyperglycaemia) have different signs and parents can learn to recognise them quickly.

Low blood sugar	High blood sugar
Trembling	Needing to urinate frequently
Sweating	Feeling very thirsty
Dizziness	Nausea
Feeling very hungry	Blurred vision
Increased heart rate	Tiredness
Anxiety	Dry mouth
	Weakness
	Irritability and tearfulness

By and large, high blood sugar is a significantly greater threat to the body than low blood sugar. Low blood sugar can be quickly remedied by ingesting a bit of glucose (e.g. a glass of apple juice): this quickly eliminates the sugar deficit and your child can go on playing right away.

It is insulin's job to bring down high blood sugar levels. However, if you are struggling to regulate your child's blood sugar levels, **seek medical advice**.

How you can help

Many parents hope that one day diabetes will be cured with homeopathy or anthroposophic medicine. Unfortunately, this is not yet possible. What is possible, however, is to provide constitutional therapy (see page 248), which generally leads to improvements in your child's overall health.

Because we are dealing with an autoimmune disorder, strengthening the activity of the 'I' in the child's metabolism is important. We recommend a twice-yearly, 2-month course of:

- Daily baths or sponge baths with rosemary bath milk.
- Phosphorus 8X, 5–10 drops in a little water in the morning.
- Rubellite 10X, 5 drops in a little water in the evening.
- Curative eurythmy (see page 242), even for babies, has also proved helpful.

Constitutional therapy

- *To unite the soul and spirit more strongly with carbohydrate and fat metabolism:* Phosphorus in higher potencies, i.e. 20X to 30X, 5 drops in the morning.
- *To improve attitude and outlook, especially in those prone to low blood sugar at night:* Hepatodoron, chew 2–3 tablets at night-time, increasing to 2 tablets 3 times a day if the single

dose is not effective enough. The effect generally becomes noticeable in the second month of treatment. Duration of treatment should be at least 3 months, followed by a 1-month break. Subsequent treatment may be either in courses with breaks or ongoing, as needed.

- *To support effective spirit and soul activity in the body:* Meteoric iron, 5 globules twice daily (morning and evening) for at least 1 month; repeat after a break as appropriate.
- *To support inner spiritual presence when restless in feelings and actions:* Oil dispersion bath with 10% rosemary etheric oil once to several times weekly. The temperature of the bath should be at least 37°C so it feels actively warm.

8.2 Type 2 diabetes

Both Type 1 and Type 2 diabetes are characterised by higher than usual blood sugar levels, but there are important differences between them. In Type 1 diabetes, the pancreas stops producing insulin, hence inhibiting the body's ability to regulate its blood sugar levels; in Type 2 diabetes, the body loses its ability to respond to insulin ('insulin resistance'), which means that the body cannot regulate blood sugar levels as well as it should. Type 2 diabetes also has different causes from Type 1 diabetes, particularly obesity and high blood pressure, and having a close relative with Type 2 diabetes means your child is more at risk of developing it. Type 2 diabetes is much less common in children than Type 1; however, Type 2 diabetes in children is on the rise.

Causes

In Western countries there has been a marked increase in the percentage of children and teenagers who are overweight or obese. Type 2 diabetes (sometimes called adult-onset diabetes) is still uncommon in children, at an incidence of less than 1%, although the disease has been increasing among children and often goes unrecognised for a long time.

The increase is related to significant lifestyle changes among children and teens in recent decades: many children get much less exercise, spend much more time sitting in front of screens, and they have a very wide range of food available to them.

The human body, however, is designed to handle a great deal of physical activity and a limited range of food. To decrease the risk of developing Type 2 diabetes, today's children need to be taught early and consciously to limit their food intake and engage in deliberate, creative physical activity. If a child is already overweight, health changes of this sort require considerable effort and are especially difficult when stress or psychiatric illnesses (e.g. ADHD, emotional disturbances, depression) are also present in the family.

Eating is one of the most fundamental needs of our existence. Physiologically, it is a response to feeling hungry that leads to enjoyment and satisfaction. The culture of eating is intimately bound up with the socialisation of children and adolescents and is associated with well-being and pleasant habitual routines. Mealtimes are places for people to share experiences, the little high and low points of the day. Eating is almost the first thing a newborn learns to do.

A balanced diet covers all the nutrients children and teens need for growth. Meals should be eaten without 'competition' from television and mobile phones. This will help your child to learn to perceive hunger, appetite and satiety appropriately.

The average time households spend on preparing meals has been significantly reduced by the introduction of ready meals and frozen foods. There is some indication that the immune system is negatively affected by the many additives in processed foods, and significant increases in autoimmune disorders and allergies may be related to this situation.

Children who are overweight can be teased by their peers, and this can make them withdraw from their social surroundings. Often they will no longer risk engaging in sports activities or even going swimming. Because of their weight, physical activity of any sort becomes slower and clumsier and takes more effort, which in turn leads to even more inactivity and social withdrawal. Lack of motivation, low self-esteem and sometimes even aggression, all of which can increase the need to eat, complete the picture.

Warning signs

- Feeling thirsty all the time
- Urinating more than usual, especially at night
- Obesity
- Tiredness
- Losing weight without trying
- Blurred vision
- High blood pressure
- Itching around the genitals or repeatedly getting thrush
- Cuts taking longer than usual to heal

Initial treatment and diabetes education

Once your child has been diagnosed, your doctor will usually prescribe medication to help lower their blood sugar (note that unlike Type 1 diabetes, insulin is often not required, although it may be in some cases) and give advice on any helpful changes to your child's diet and activity. Your child will need to have regular check-ups and you will be educated about the signs of related health problems that could develop in the future (e.g. heart disease, stroke, foot infections, vision loss, kidney problems, and numbness and pain).

Although the consequences of Type 2 diabetes can be managed, treating it is a lifelong effort. Repeated short-term weight-loss diets are not an effective solution to Type 1 diabetes. Obesity programmes that are designed for the long term – at least 1 year – and involve the whole family have better chances of success.

How you can help

One of the key aims of treating Type 2 diabetes is assisting with weight loss. If your child is overweight, the support of the whole family can be a great help. If your entire family can rethink their habits around food and physical activity and acquire new ones, it will make things much easier for the diabetic child.

Fundamental lifestyle changes, such as increased physical activity, serving smaller portions of food, relearning the culture of eating and reducing media consumption are important first steps that will have long-term benefits for your child, yourself and the whole family. Shared activities such as regular hikes are both helpful and enjoyable.

Complementary anthroposophic therapies are recommended but need to be prescribed individually, e.g. curative eurythmy (see page 242), along with anthroposophic medicines. Ask your doctor for advice.

9. Cancer

There have been major changes and developments in paediatric oncology in the last 50 years. New connections have been discovered in basic research and new forms of therapy developed in clinical practice. Today, childhood cancers can often be completely cured, thanks to the tireless commitment of many doctors and patients involved in studies.

In the UK, 1,600 cases of childhood cancer (children aged 0–14) are diagnosed every year. However, whereas 50 years ago only 25% of children diagnosed with cancer survived, today the average 5-year survival rate across all childhood cancers is 82%. In some types of cancer the percentages are even higher: for example, the survival rate from eye cancer (retinoblastoma) is now 100%; from lymphoma, 91%; and from leukaemia, 89%.[4]

These statistics represent a clear success for modern medicine. **Therefore children with cancer should be treated according to standardised therapeutic protocols**, which consist almost without exception of chemotherapy and in some cases surgery and/or radiation therapy. The protocols are routinely re-evaluated and modified to improve the prognosis still further and reduce side effects.

How do we recognise cancer in a child?

Often a cluster of several symptoms lead medical professionals to consider cancer in a child. These may include:
- Lumps or swellings
- Lasting pain
- Unusual sweating
- Lasting headaches or dizziness
- Tiredness
- Sudden weight loss
- Unexplained bruising or bleeding

For example, the symptoms of leukaemia might include lasting fatigue, headache and weakness, along with little areas of bleeding within the skin or unexplainable bruises. Swollen lymph nodes, bone pain or, in toddlers, conspicuous unwillingness to walk or move can also suggest a malignancy. The first indications of a brain tumour may be headaches associated with poor coordination, paralysis, visual blackouts, and nausea and vomiting in the morning.

If your child has symptoms that might suggest a malignancy, it is imperative that you discuss them with your doctor. Often the concern turns out to be unfounded. If warranted, your doctor will order a blood test or other diagnostic measures.

Even though childhood cancer is rare, many parents are understandably afraid of their child having cancer, especially if they have persistent, indeterminate symptoms of illness. Fortunately, as the figures cited above indicate, this applies to very few families.

However, sometimes parents' fears are realised and their child is diagnosed with cancer. A cancer diagnosis can throw all members of the family off track, and they must all come to grips with it. For parents and the wider family, life will now be dominated by the shock of the diagnosis, concern for their child and the fear of possibly losing them. Although it can seem overwhelming to imagine telling friends and rela-

tives about your child's diagnosis, many parents find it helpful to share their news. Informing family and friends about the child's illness and treatment can make it easier for them to offer support and empathy.

Causes

When a child is diagnosed with cancer, parents have many questions, for example: 'Why our child? What did we do wrong? And what caused the cancer?'

Tumours and leukaemia are fundamentally different from other diseases because in the great majority of cases, with the exception of radiation accidents and atomic catastrophes, they cannot be traced back to anything that comes from outside. Rather, the illness involves the child's constitution and destiny. The problem that manifests as the illness comes from within. Therefore it makes more sense to avoid looking for external causes and how they might have been eliminated or suppressed. Instead, we might ask: 'How can we help the child to curb the tumour-producing tendency?'

Anthroposophic treatment

To complement the child's treatment with conventional medicine, it is essential to support their healthy life forces, emotional balance and individuality with a view to increasing their autonomy and forces of resistance. Anthroposophic paediatric oncology goes beyond the conventional therapeutic protocol on three levels:

- *1. Bodily level:* Anthroposophic medicines and the external application of wraps, compresses, rubs and massages help patients' bodies. Central to anthroposophic treatment is mistletoe therapy, which is believed to slow tumour growth and improve quality of life. It can be administered either by injection under the skin in the area of the tumour or as oral drops. This treatment has been used in paediatric cancer cases for many years at the general hospital in Herdecke and there are also scientific studies and numerous case studies supporting the use of this therapy. Significant side effects are not expected if mistletoe therapy is implemented correctly, although fever and local reactions are desirable because they indicate that the immune system is being stimulated.
- *2. Soul level:* Artistic therapies awaken children's creative potential and transform the destructive ones.
- *3. Biographical level:* Through questions directed primarily to the parents of children with cancer to ascertain what may be developed to prevent a recurrence.

One study showed that anthroposophic medicine played a significant role in paediatric oncology in Germany. Nearly 75% of anthroposophic treatments were prescribed by a doctor, versus only about 35% of other complementary treatments. 90% of parents had discussed integrating anthroposophic medicine into conventional treatment. 18% opted for anthroposophic constitutional therapy and 16% for the mistletoe products. Of these, approximately 96% of parents surveyed would recommend this type of treatment to others as a complement to conventional medicine.[5]

Conventional therapeutic models generally do not consider these aspects. Affected children remain the passive victims of their altered, damaged genes, so to speak, and can only let it all wash over them.

We find it important to speak on all levels to the child's healthy forces and possibilities and to rouse them to do battle against the cancer (see also page 236 for more on salutogenesis). This allows not only children but also their parents to make a contribution towards either their cure or towards living with the disease, as the case may be.

Childhood cancer, however, has social significance in addition to these individual aspects. Reports from affected parents show that they experienced issues of meaning, whether present or future-directed, as very helpful and comforting, opening up new perspectives, ways forwards and options for dealing with this stroke of destiny. As time goes on, the child's illness may even reveal a unique meaning or purpose all of its own. Many parents report changes of this sort, and once a little distance is achieved the illness can suddenly appear in a different light.

Although childhood cancers remain life-threatening diseases, modern treatments enable cures in most cases. Accompanying young people through this phase of the illness, both bodily and emotionally, is especially important, because a child who comes to grips with a life-threatening illness at an early age will carry this experience with them for a lifetime, in body but more particularly in soul (see also Chapter 15, Facing Tough Challenges). The most essential thing, therefore, is to help the child cultivate enjoyment of life and hope for their future.

10. Mental Health

10.1 Emotional pain

Children of all ages experience many different types of emotional pain, which mark the beginning of the part of a child's biography that is the shadow side of the good and happy experiences. Children may demonstrate any of the following behaviours:

- They may cry bitterly or become anxious when they know their parents plan to go out in the evening.
- They may feel unjustly treated or react emotionally to punishment at the hands of their parents or caregivers.
- They may feel themselves caught in conflicts between their parents.
- They may become outsiders in school or kindergarten, be excluded from their classmates' friendships and cliques, or even be subjected to bullying.
- They may be teased because of their clothes, appearance or disabilities.
- If they are older, they may be subject to pangs of conscience or feelings of shame, profound grief, hopelessness or despair.

Emotional pain is always an indication of separation, a sign that the psyche has been prevented from participating harmoniously in its surroundings or revealing itself freely and gladly to its companions.

Such pain has a much more profound effect on children than on adults, in spite of the fact that some adults tend to imagine that children have no real problems at all. Adults, after all, can distance themselves from problems by processing them and thinking them through, while children cannot. The younger they are, the more direct the effect of events around them. Their suffering is uniquely intense because they do not really understand it and cannot let go of it.

If such suffering is associated with injury and experiencing violence, trauma can be extensive. Trauma therapies have become established worldwide since the

1970s, and can offer a great deal of information and insight.

Watch particularly if children become increasingly quiet. The only immediate help you can offer these children is to distract them and help them to forget.

Conversation with an adult can help an older child process emotional pain, but a great deal depends on the adult's response to the event that triggered it. One-sided expressions of sympathy or tirades against the event do not help. It is helpful, however, if the adult can convey to the child (either with or without words) that their deep suffering has been perceived and taken seriously. (See also Chapter 15, Facing Tough Challenges).

Before the age of 10, children are not yet able to objectively process emotional crises or the aftermath of traumatic events. But if they feel that an adult is attempting to deal with their problem, acknowledging it rather than ignoring it, they can sense that their pain does have some kind of meaning. They can feel that although bad things happen, they happen within a larger, living, breathing context and are familiar and manageable to adults.

For example, if a child tormented by anxiety has contact with an adult who has achieved a profound trust in destiny, the longing to do likewise is implanted, consciously or unconsciously, in the child's soul. Later on, this child will more easily learn to overcome their anxious approach to the world.

Something we have already noted with regard to dealing with physical pain is also true of emotional pain. It is up to adults to consciously carry, process and overcome that part of the burden that a child cannot yet come to grips with. Ultimately, the universal remedy for all types of emotional pain is warm, authentic interest in the person affected by it; in other words, our own understanding and love.

10.2 Fear and anxiety

Most of us will have been amazed at toddlers who, without the slightest hesitation, will climb up a ladder or stand at the edge of a cliff, but this existential fearlessness can disappear from one moment to the next if they are awakened by a bad dream or a loud crash, experience traumatic pain or are forced to watch someone being abused. The most common cause, however, is feeling abandoned. Anxiety sets in and becomes their constant companion, posing a question and a challenge to the adults around them.

Some children (and some adults) use such events to become stronger, while others must first feed their fears. People who tend to distance themselves from events and prefer to have everything explained, planned and thoroughly considered are usually more anxious than hands-on types and enthusiastic experimenters.

Of course how we *are* as adults, not how we would like to be, is what affects children. Parents are often afraid that their children might be afraid of the doctor, yet pre-emptive assurances like 'You don't have to be afraid of the doctor' are more likely to trigger fears than calm them. We have found that visits to the doctor can be especially traumatic for children raised in institutions, who often panic during examinations or when blood has to be drawn. This is a sign of the extent to which lack of human love and attention during the first few years of life disrupts the development of healthy self-confidence.

Treating fears and anxieties is one of the greatest tasks not only of psychiatry, psychotherapy and medicine as a whole, but also of pastoral counselling. Conversation, understanding, the passage of time and medication are all helpful.

In general, acknowledging and accepting fear is the first step towards overcoming it. Your physical presence, time and brief, objective comments will help your child combat fear, but long speeches will not. Distracting children's attention from their own anxious thoughts to real, understandable perceptions helps even more. Make it possible for your child to get to know people who are not afraid or who have learned to manage their fear.

Fear has an important defence function on both physical and emotional levels. It awakens, makes one aware and strengthens self-observation. It can be a lifelong task to work at keeping fear within healthy boundaries. The body is vulnerable and susceptible to dangers from both outside and within. Only the eternal part of human beings, their spiritual essence, is indestructible and eternal. The more we become conscious of this, the easier it is to put our fears into perspective. However, there are fears that many children hold in common and we can offer a few tips on dealing with these:

Fear of thunderstorms

Hold your child while you watch the lightning together and comment on the loudness of the thunderclaps. When they calm down a bit, comment on the lightning flashes, saying things like, 'See how bright that one is!' or (later) 'Look, how pretty!' – but only if you yourself can truly appreciate its beauty. Children older than 9 can understand the statement, 'If you heard the thunder, it means the lightning didn't strike you,' but the reason this is soothing to them is less because of its logic than because they realise you are capable of commenting calmly on what you both perceive.

Fear of drawing blood

The best preparation is to hold your child and tell them, 'I'll hold you, and the doctor will tell us what he's going to do.' This establishes the doctor's authority while also making your child feel physically protected.

Imaginary fears

Being afraid of a man in black or a dark cellar is usually based on silly talk or snatches of conversation children have heard. They may develop similarly unfounded fears if they hear themselves described as 'afraid of the water', 'dizzy' or even just 'shy'. Thoughts like these tend to mushroom in children's imaginations, but they will proudly disprove these statements (away

from the person who makes them) if a trusted companion accompanies them into a dark room, into the water or to the edge of a cliff.

10.3 Anorexia nervosa

Anorexia is a psychogenic eating disorder characterised by disturbed body image, distorted and fixed ideas about food intake, pathological fear of gaining weight and failure to recognise the condition as an illness. This disorder appears only in the modern industrial world. Although the number of cases among boys is increasing, the overwhelming majority of people with anorexia are teenage girls and young women. Excessive weight loss is accompanied by absence of menstruation and, in most cases, constipation. These young women are often athletic and scholastic high-achievers, and many of them enjoy gourmet cooking and feeding others. On the whole, these patients appear compulsive; their thoughts always revolve around food, calories, their weight and their figures, and often around purity and transgression as well. They implement strategies that lead to physical deterioration and disrupt their development; weight loss may be so extreme that it becomes life-threatening.

Experts agree that the self-assertive, defiant phase of early childhood and the successful establishment of self-identity after the so-called 'rubicon' of the tenth year are absent from these young women's biographies. No general links can be made to family ranking or parent–child relationships. As with other psychological disorders in childhood, there is some correlation with early experiences of physical abuse.

In spite of many psychological and social attempts to define this illness, it always presents new riddles. Because of the age of the majority of anorexia patients, puberty was formerly thought to be a triggering factor, but this interpretation conceals the patients' underlying mistrust in the body as a whole as the 'house of the soul'. The illness presents a difficult therapeutic challenge in that the goal of therapy is to rebuild the entire basis for the life of the physical body. In addition to special diets and intravenous feeding (if necessary) and anthroposophic and naturopathic medications, external treatments in the form of compresses and ointments (see page 293) are indicated to stimulate and strengthen the senses of life, touch and warmth. These initial treatments can soon be followed by artistic therapies such as painting, curative eurythmy or music therapy. Later, speech therapy and Bothmer gymnastics are appropriate. Individual and family psychotherapy sessions foster maturation of the patient's personality and increase receptivity to their social surroundings.

11. ADHD
and Dyslexia

In the past, children with behavioural and learning disorders were simply considered fidgety and were marginalised for their 'naughty' behaviour. Today, however, we know that they suffer from constitutional disorders for which neither they nor their parents can be held morally accountable. Only one thing is important: to understand each child's particular situation and do what we can to help.

11.1 Attention deficit and hyperactivity disorder (ADHD)

We all know children who appear restless and driven, act impulsively, are difficult to engage in conversation and react to even mild or imagined disruptions with aggression. These children have difficulty making connections between thoughts. Their excessive expressions of sympathy and antipathy and frequently destructive behaviour are often not met with understanding. In spite of widely varying symptoms, children with ADHD have one thing in common: the inability to pay attention and control their impulses, hence the name 'attention deficit and hyperactivity disorder'.

Hyperactivity is sometimes complicated by the presence of other disorders, such as nervous tics. Hyperactive children may also have specific learning difficulties, like dyslexia, isolated writing disorders, problems understanding what they hear or listening when several people are speaking at the same time. **Thorough examination and diagnosis by a child psychiatrist or experienced specialist paediatrician is an important first step in dealing with the problem.**

Causes

A combination of factors is thought to contribute to the causes of ADHD, though these are not yet fully understood. Genetics is thought to play a part, because ADHD tends to run in families. Brain structure may also contribute: some studies suggest that in people with ADHD some areas of the brain may be smaller and some larger than those without ADHD. There are also groups who are believed to be more at risk of ADHD, such as:

- People who were born prematurely.
- People with epilepsy.
- People with brain damage.

Symptoms

ADHD can be split into two types of behavioural problems: inattentiveness and hyperactivity. If you child has ADHD they may have symptoms that cover both of these categories, but not always (see box on Attention Deficit Disorder). **It is important to consult your doctor in order to get an accurate diagnosis.**

Symptoms of inattentiveness

- Short attention span
- Easily distracted
- Forgetfulness
- Carelessness
- Being unable to finish tasks that are time-consuming or boring
- Seeming unable to listen or carry out instructions
- Difficulty organising tasks

Symptoms of hyperactivity

- Constant fidgeting
- Unable to sit still (especially in quiet surroundings) and excessive movement
- Lack of concentration
- Interrupting and excessive talking
- Acting without thinking
- Lack of awareness of danger

Attention deficit disorder (ADD)

Attention deficit disorder (ADD) can sometimes be confused with ADHD. Children with ADD have difficulties with concentration but not necessarily with impulsiveness or hyperactivity. Typical symptoms are those associated with inattentiveness (see below), but a key feature of ADD is daydreaming or children being distracted by their own thoughts. As with ADHD, it is essential to see your doctor for a diagnosis.

Treatment

From the anthroposophic perspective, this cluster of symptoms deals with the mastery of the individual's 'I' over his or her soul life. Attention and concentration, emotional balance and readiness to act, are all inadequately controlled in a child with ADHD. When developing a treatment plan, therefore, it is important to answer the following questions:

- Who are the adults who have, or will acquire, the strength and ability to understand, empathise with and stand by this child?
- How can we reduce and, if possible, eliminate the factors in daily life that intensify the child's symptoms?
- Where can we find an experienced special needs education specialist who will provide the needed individual time and attention for the child, and support for teachers and parents? It is important that treatment or self-help begins as early as possible.
- Will we resort to treating the child with stimulants such as methylphenidate (Ritalin) and others, which has become the standard treatment worldwide?

Low doses of medications such as Ritalin (methylphenidate) have calming and attention-enhancing effects on most hyperactive children, and the effects last for several hours. Amphetamines (performance-enhancing stimulants that are also used as appetite suppressants) have similar effects. So does coffee, although its effects are weaker. Reports from enthusiastic children, parents and teachers indicate that taking medications such as Ritalin produce sudden and dramatic improvement in many children's situations in school and at home. It is said that in the US, 10% of all boys are treated with Ritalin; in Mexico City, the figure is 30%.

We recommend three means of treating the causes of ADHD:

1. Are there any aspects of the child's environment and lifestyle that tend to increase symptoms? Reduce or, wherever possible, eliminate these.
2. Early directed special needs education, consisting of individual training to strengthen the control function of the child sense of self, the 'I', has been very successful.
3. Medical treatment with anthroposophic or homeopathic constitutional remedies.

If unavoidable, temporary professional treatment with Ritalin or similar stimulants can be helpful as a short-term measure.

The remainder of this section will deal with aids that may be used in individual cases as needed and as the circumstances permit.

Cooperative conversation

If it is possible to arrange, we encourage a cooperative conversation between everybody involved in educating and treating the child: for example, parents, caregivers and teachers, as well as the child's doctor, therapist(s) and other important people in the child's life. In the course of this conversation, each person should present a personal image of the child and their talents and possibilities. The collective image is then filled out by characterising both the child's learning difficulties and their abilities and strengths as exactly as possible. Interim objectives and long-term treatment goals should be considered. Tasks should be assigned to the participants, any necessary helpers enlisted, and regular reviews scheduled. It is essential for the child to participate in developing very concrete strategies to overcome each specific difficulty, because nothing will work without strong motivation. These strategies should be fun and lead to successful experiences.

A rhythmical daily routine

Hyperactive children need firm, reasonable, externally imposed routines for every day of the week. The adults around the child must know the child's exact daily and weekly schedule, be aware of less frequent but regular events, and know who is responsible for the child and when. Even the first few minutes after waking up and the last moments before falling asleep need to be specially structured. A bedtime ritual can become a highlight of your child's day. After hearing a brief story and singing a song, exchange a few words about how the day went. What happened today? What will happen tomorrow? A mood of quiet observation and positivity is best. Complete the ritual with a song, a prayer or a beautiful verse. This routine helps your child 'digest' both food and the day's events.

Your morning greeting should also be lighthearted, full of warm humour and should radiate certainty that a successful day at school lies ahead for your child.

Visual aids

Children with ADHD often have a problem connecting spoken words with meaningful actions. A written daily and weekly plan is helpful because they are better able to connect to a visual statement.

Physical activity

Hyperactive children need to walk to school. 20–30 minutes of walking will help them to stay in their seats in school – and please their teachers. Afternoons at home (or at a neighbour's or at a nearby farm) should also include plenty of opportunities for physical activity: gardening, sawing wood, helping with the wheelbarrow, woodwork and other crafts, or going on half-day hikes with the family or school groups.

No electronic media

Television, phones, music players and devices that allow internet access should disappear from your child's immediate surroundings. Even in constitutionally healthy children, early and frequent media consumption causes obvious damage that manifests as attention deficits and inability to listen or grasp connections. Media consumption can significantly increase symptoms of hyperactivity and thus make your child's overall situation worse. Once your child is 10 or 11 years old, you and your child can select a limited number of programmes or films to watch, but always watch them together and discuss them afterwards.

Living space

We recommend putting away everything you don't absolutely need. Use heavy ceramic tumblers and mugs that can't tip over easily. Instead of candle holders (which can tip over and get blown out), use lanterns with tea lights. Place a footstool under the table so your child has something solid to rest their feet on. Small rooms with doors that close are better than

large, open-plan, multi-purpose areas. When your child is helping in a shop or in the kitchen, have them stand on a low stool: the need for balance and the slight change in perspective will increase their attentiveness.

Nutrition

Phosphates, glutamates, flavour-enhancers, food colouring, and preservatives as well as a number of possible food allergies have been implicated in symptoms of hyperactivity. We do not advise special low-phosphate diets because some very important foods such as milk and nuts contain phosphates. We do, however, recommend a healthy, grain-based diet (including less common grains, such as spelt, millet, buckwheat and quinoa) with adequate amounts of salad and fruit. We suggest emphasising vegetarian meals or moderating meat consumption.

Any foods that you suspect of increasing your child's symptoms should be eliminated temporarily and then reintroduced one at a time in small (initially imperceptible) amounts mixed in with other foods. Give your child the newly reintroduced food every other day, and gradually increase the amounts until you notice restlessness. Leave the amount the same while you watch to see if your child gets used to it. Your goal is to allow your child to eat as wide a variety of foods as possible.

No form of testing can be considered an adequate substitute for your child actually trying out foods. In the case of sweets, begin with raisins and other dried fruits and then move on to good-quality honey, small amounts of evaporated cane juice and even white sugar in very small quantities, for sweetening yoghurt and the like. We do not recommend ready-made sweetened products because they all contain far too much sugar. In our experience, chocolate and foods containing cocoa powder are also not good.

If your child becomes unusually restless after eating a home-made dessert, don't break off the experiment immediately. Instead, say, 'We'll try that again the day after tomorrow.' This gives your child an opportunity to see if they can control their restlessness. Do not do this kind of challenge testing just before school, however, because it sets your child up for disappointment.

One experienced child psychiatrist recommends giving school-age children a cup of coffee in the morning. This may seem unlikely but, like Ritalin therapy, it has been shown to have a calming effect.

Sensory education

By this we mean education of all the sensory functions described in this book (see page 237). Especially important for hyperactive children are the senses of touch, balance, movement (kinaesthesia) and life, which transmit sensations of one's own body. Rhythmical patterns of sleeping, waking and eating are especially important. Sensory education is part of all the therapeutic and educational measures discussed below.

Kindergarten

Choosing the right kindergarten can provide significant respite for parents. However, avoid placing your hyperactive child in a large-group setting or an understaffed programme, as this can lead to early experiences of failure and marginalisation. Already at this age, arranging the above-mentioned cooperative conversation among all concerned adults and implementing the relevant conclusions can be a great help to your child's further development.

School

In a school setting, a hyperactive child's problems become much more apparent. Small classes or smaller subgroups in large classes are very helpful. (In defence of teachers, it should be noted that even one or two hyperactive children in a large class can wreck the most carefully prepared lesson.) Here, too, if possible, it is important to begin conversations with your child's teacher before problems arise, to establish mutual trust and lines of communication. For example, if your child has been horse-riding and you noticed that your restless child became very quiet and attentive because of the subconscious effort required to maintain balance, the unconventional step of providing a large gymnastic ball or a bar stool for him to sit on whenever he gets restless in class may be very helpful. If deftly managed, this adaptive measure signals to the class that restlessness is a natural occurrence for this child and not something that merits much attention. To the hyperactive child, it signals that they can be confident in their teacher's desire to help them. This and other such helpful measures work well, however, only if good contact has been established among all involved with the child.

Sensory integration therapy

Sensory integration therapy exposes children to sensory stimulation in a structured way, to help them deal with sensory processing issues. Along with physical therapy, it is always recommended if a child has difficulty integrating their perceptions and actions.

Occupational therapy

This can begin at home with parents: for example, painting, using modelling clay and braiding. Slightly more difficult activities could include simple hand weaving or stitching with a blunt darning needle. If a workshop is available, your child should learn to hammer, to split wood with a wedge and especially to saw (with a parent helping to guide the saw). If these opportunities are not available at home, look for a professional occupational therapist who can provide them.

Special education and behavioural therapy

Therapy sessions with an educational specialist or behavioural psychologist can be limited to once or twice a week. As long-term treatments, they are very successful if the practitioner is experienced.

Parental training

This offers parents educational help using elements of behavioural therapy. They learn to cope with typical everyday problems independently and learn to better understand their child and his special nature.

Singing and music therapy

Singing cultivates the emotional forces that can be suppressed by uncontrolled feelings if they are left to their own devices. The Nordoff Robbins improvisational model of music therapy attempts to express in music the movements a child is making at the moment, thus conveying to them on a semi-conscious level that they are understood and accompanied. Its benefits include stimulating attentiveness and reducing problems at home.

Storytelling and speech

A daily 'story hour' adapted to your child's age and level of understanding can work wonders. Read aloud to your child in a calm, natural, not overly dramatic tone of voice.

Rhythmical massage

The technique of rhythmic 'einreibung', as developed by Ita Wegman (see page 77), can help children to feel comfortable in their body and control it better.

Bothmer gymnastics

Although still relatively unknown, this is excellent for developing a good body image. It was introduced in the first Waldorf school, and since that time, therapeutic applications have been developed specifically for hyperactive children and teens with eating disorders.

Curative eurythmy

Adapted for use with children, curative eurythmy aids self-discovery by strengthening the movements of both body and soul (see page 242).

External applications

Compresses, baths and oil rubs administered for secondary health problems, or as additional stimulating or calming measures, can help hyperactive children in a variety of ways. They are generally prescribed by experienced physicians or therapists.

11.2 Dyslexia

Dyslexia is understood as an isolated learning disorder that affects reading and writing and appears in otherwise normally intelligent children. Approximately 3–8% of children are affected. Parents and teachers can provide effective assistance to children and help them to avoid unnecessary suffering. In this section, we will attempt to present a few perspectives that will aid in understanding and managing this condition.

Symptoms
Preschool children

- Speech problems, e.g. jumbling up letters in phrases and struggling to pronounce long words
- Delayed speech development
- Problems with expression, e.g. not remembering the right word
- Lack of interest in and understanding of rhymes and learning the alphabet

Primary school children

- Difficulties learning the names and sounds of letters
- Difficulties learning sequences (e.g. the alphabet) and carrying out a sequence of instructions
- Putting letters and numbers the wrong way around, e.g. 'd' instead of 'b' and vice versa
- Poor and slow handwriting
- Inconsistent spelling and confusing the order of letters
- Reading slowly and making mistakes when reading aloud
- Difficulty writing down answers to questions but answering well orally
- Poor phonological awareness and difficulty breaking up words into phonological parts

Understanding dyslexia

To learn to write words, children must be able and willing to extract individual sounds from a word they know only as a whole: i.e. to break the word down into parts. Instead of paying attention to its meaning, they are now supposed to focus exclusively on specific, isolated sounds. At the same time, a second abstraction is demanded of them: to believe that an arbitrary symbol is the sound itself. Until this point, children have believed they are able to 'read' an upside-down picture book. Try to imagine what it means when they are suddenly confronted with these qualitatively equivalent and meaningless symbols:

These abstract characters made of straight and curved lines acquire meaning only through a very specific spatial relationship to the reader, and they can't even be pronounced without adding a vowel. For children, being asked to recreate words from such imprecise characters is a truly impenetrable art. Why is the vowel in 'the' an *e* instead of a *u*? Why do we write 'h-e-r-e' or 'h-e-a-r' instead of 'h-e-r'?

We hope these examples make it clear how easy it is for uncertainty and confusion to arise. Children who still try to interpret letters as pictures will have trouble, as will those who take their teachers' statements too literally when told to 'spell it the way it sounds'. Already at this point, it should be obvious that teaching reading and writing in child-friendly ways takes quite a long time. Equally obviously, the teacher must know all the details that can trip up dyslexics and be able to separate the process of learning to write into small, manageable steps based on phonetic research.

Remarkably, some children learn to write and read almost by themselves, and mastering all the exceptions to phonetic rules comes as easily as playing. It is as if they simply have to 'remember' how to write. For others, however, their world falls apart. Although they might be used to having minimal difficulties, or none at all, with spatial orientation and doing whatever their peers do, now all of a sudden they are being asked to do something that remains totally unfathomable to them. For a while, they write according to laws that dyslexia experts recognise as derived from especially good attempts to listen. Later, however, as they become increasingly resigned to failure, their written words become increasingly distorted.

At this point, symptoms such as pallor, susceptibility to infec-tion, fatigue, listlessness, insomnia, stomachaches, wetting and aggression often appear. The list of complaints that eventually lead unrecognised dyslexics to the doctor's office even includes serious physical illnesses. Even then, the fact that dyslexia is either causing or contributing to their symptoms is easily overlooked. The appearance of physical and psychological symptoms, however, is a clear sign that the condition needs to be treated as an illness. Obviously, it is not enough to base a diagnosis of dyslexia on the fact that a child confuses d with b or p with q.

Meanwhile, other deficits might have developed, and their causes are more difficult to assess. **Thorough diagnosis by a doctor, followed by individual help and support is required.** Not only the child's writing errors but also their general spatial orientation, control over their body, perception of forms and their ability to speak and understand speech must be analysed in detail before deciding on an individual treatment plan. As soon as the child begins to experience some success as a result of therapy and the first signs of progress become visible, their confidence will grow and physical symptoms will soon disappear.

How you can help

Adequate time must be allowed for special needs support with writing and reading to be fully effective: 1–2 years if the problem is recognised early and approached holistically, usually longer if it is not. For severe cases, we recommend contacting a programme specialising in dyslexia therapy. Sensory-motor integration therapy and/or curative eurythmy also help increase the chance of success. In all cases, however, close cooperation among therapists, teachers, and parents is necessary.

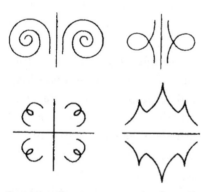

Examples of symmetry exercises for walking or drawing.

Toddlers who seem clumsy, sleepy or slow to learn to talk can be helped by encouraging their sensory activity and memory, and by structuring the course of the day and year rhythmically (see page 244). Stimulation of this sort supports the necessary metamorphosis of growth forces into thought forces. This transformation, which is irregular in cases of dyslexia, is the prerequisite of any kind of thought activity.

In the first few years of school, children who have trouble orienting themselves in space, time and their own consciousness can benefit from measures implemented during school hours by teachers or therapists:

- Perception exercises: observing and describing the shapes of objects together. Pictures, plants or stones can be used.
- Walking shapes and their mirror images on the floor.
- Drawing the forms with their feet, holding thick crayons between their toes.
- Drawing the forms in the air with their hands, keeping their eyes closed.
- Repeating the process the next day, then helping the children to visualise it and finally drawing the forms on paper.
- Repeating all of the above steps (with the exception of the symmetry exercises) using letter shapes.
- Exercises in writing what they hear, beginning with the simplest syllables. Playful but systematic transition to multi-syllable words with

phonetic spellings and only later to words that require knowing spelling rules.

- Later, writing short texts from dictation. To maximise success, all of the words selected for this purpose should be spelled the way they sound.
- Curative eurythmy treatments, where available.

There are corresponding techniques for children with difficulties with maths.

When dealing with dyslexic children, it is important to convey a happy and optimistic attitude, because their problems are often intensified by a sense of failure and either inadequate moral support or resignation on the part of adults. It is possible to support dyslexic children very effectively, and many learn to read and write well.

12. Babies and Young Children

Parents recalling their first child's first day of life often say they knew that everything would be different from then on. No amount of preparation for the birth of a child can even approximate the experience of how profoundly this little being, in all their helplessness, moves and shapes the feelings, thoughts, and actions of those around them.

12.1 Some questions about birth

Should I be concerned about giving birth in hospital?

The options for delivery today range from home births through to outpatient or inpatient delivery in the obstetrics department of a hospital (with or without an in-house neonatal clinic) to highly specialised perinatal centres for 'high-risk' births.

In some areas, efforts have gone into making hospital births as comfortable and intimate as traditional home birthing, with technological devices being kept in the background to avoid a cold and impersonal atmosphere. The birthing team accompanies the event discreetly, with a surgical team and a paediatrician close by in case of emergency.

If there are medical reasons for a hospital delivery or if a hospital birth simply feels safer and more comfortable to you, it's a good idea to check that your baby will stay in the room with you at all times (provided specialist care is not required). In the first few days, it is important for mother and child to spend as much time together as possible in order to develop their connection. In most birthing clinics, fathers are integrated into caring for the baby to a considerable extent. They are allowed to support the mother before and during birth and share instruction in caring for the newborn if they so desire.

If there have been indications during the pregnancy that the newborn may require hospital care for a while – for example, if the baby is premature or their birth weight low – it makes sense to give birth in a hospital with both obstetric and neonatal departments to avoid unnecessary separation during the first few days.

Post-birth preventative measures

Supplemental Vitamin K

Vitamin K helps blood to clot. All babies are born with low levels of vitamin K, though there is usually enough to stop bleeding. However, a minority of babies (1 in 10,000) can have vitamin K deficiency bleeding (VKBD), which can be very serious – even fatal. Therefore in a number of countries, including the UK and USA, almost all midwives and obstetric clinics recommend administering vitamin K immediately after birth to prevent possible haemorrhaging, and this can be done either by injection or orally.

Among healthy infants, breast-fed babies are at greater risk if they do not receive supplementation because the vitamin K content of breast milk is very low compared to commercial formula. Children with diseases involving bile flow disorders (cholestasis) are the main risk group and need special attention. Children who require intramuscular administration of vitamin K include: full-term infants in poor overall health, children with absorption disorders and premature babies with birth weights under 1500 g (3 lb 4 oz). At the Herdecke hospital we administer an initial dose of 2 mg at birth, followed by smaller daily doses.

Stimulating coagulation processes constitutes a profound intervention in a very delicately regulated balance. Rudolf Steiner calls this the balance between albuminising and antimonising forces, related to the balance between thinking and the will. Against this background, reinforcing the coagulation side of the balance with vitamins could lead to a weakening of the will, leading into intensified conceptualisation. On this level, the significance for a newborn baby has not been adequately clarified.

Silver nitrate eye drops

In many hospitals, especially in the USA, antibiotic ointment is administered to newborns to prevent gonococcal conjunctivitis. This infection, picked up from the mother's vagina, has become uncommon in industrialized nations. The conjunctivitis can be treated effectively if caught in time, so in our opinion antibiotics should be reserved for therapeutic use if needed.

Premature babies and ill newborns

Babies born before the 35th week of gestation (premature babies, or 'preemies'), as well as some full-term babies, may require intensive care immediately after birth or during the first few days of life. In such instances, it is not always possible to avoid separating mother and child for a short time. It's a good idea to ask whether the mother can also be admitted to the neonatal unit or alternatively whether she can have a room nearby. Nowadays visiting hours are usually not strictly specified or cover many hours during the day. Parents are allowed to get to know and take care of their themselves by the baby's bedside.

Almost all neonatal intensive care units promptly place the baby in the 'kangaroo position', where they are allowed to spend many hours resting on the ribcage of their half-reclining mother or father having skin-to-skin contact. In this way, the baby feels the parent's heartbeat and breathing, which usually not only has a calming effect but also stimulates the infant's respiration. Many babies treated this way need less supplemental oxygen. Breastfeeding is usually not possible for babies in the acute stages of illness, but as soon as they are better they are given the first pumped breast milk or allowed to nurse, because colostrum is especially valuable for premature infants. Increasingly, even small preemies are encouraged to nurse.

It is becoming more common for newborns and preemies to be bedded in 'nests', even in incubators, that provide a tactile sense of enclosure, and to cover the incubators to protect the babies from exposure to the sensory overload of excessively bright lights.

12.2 The cradle and lying position

The cradle

For your baby's bed, we recommend a basket or cradle completely lined with a single-colour fabric and covered with a pale pink-violet veil. The veil keeps out irritating draughts and admits a pleasantly dimmed light conducive to peaceful sleep. If the cradle is located near an open window, the veil prevents sun from falling directly on to the baby. Of course it also blocks ultraviolet light, a consideration when light is needed to prevent rickets. In this case, pull the veil back so that direct sunlight is still mainly blocked but the baby's head is exposed to blue sky. It doesn't matter whether you use a home-made frame with rockers, an antique cradle, or any other type of movable baby basket or cradle, but it must fit beside your own bed. Parents often don't think of this, and as a result parents have to get out of bed countless times each night.

The best mattress for a baby's bed is a one-piece, flat mattress that is well filled, preferably with natural materials. The baby does not need a pillow.

Lying position

From carrying newborn babies, we know that they cannot yet hold their heads and torsos upright against the force of gravity. Only when lying on their stomachs are they able to hold their heads up briefly. Less obvious is the fact that gravity can actively deform a baby's body during the first months of life. A baby who always turns their head to the same side (towards the light or towards approaching people, for example) develops a flat area on the skull on that side. This deformation may extend all the way down the torso to the pelvis. If recognised only after the third month, this position-inflicted damage cannot be fully corrected. To prevent this deformity, alternate the side on which you position of the baby's head. If a head deformity has

already developed, your doctor may advise you to turn the head consistently toward the neglected side for a while.

If your baby can turn her head by herself and prefers the brighter side, for example, you will have to turn her (or her bed) around so that her feet are where her head used to be and the light falls on her from the other side.

Other possible reasons for preferring one side over the other include broken collarbone at birth (see page 207), muscular torticollis (wryneck, see page 208), or a swelling on the baby's head.* When either wryneck or a swelling on the head is the cause of the preference for one side, these cases need to be discussed with your doctor.

Sleeping positions: back, side or stomach?

According to more recent studies, the stomach position for infants that American experts used to advocate in the sixties contributed significantly to the increase in sudden infant death (SIDS, see

---

* A caput succedaneum (a swelling that forms on the presenting part of the foetus during delivery) disappears after a day or two, but a haematoma (a mass of clotted blood resulting from a broken vessel) recedes only after several weeks or months. It is better not to lay an infant on that side until the haematoma has resolved.

page 214). At present, the general recommendation is to put infants to sleep on their backs, not on their sides or stomachs, with no pillow. If the baby has a soft skull or begins to develop a flat spot on the back of his head, a home-made pillow, 20 x 20 cm (8 x 8 in) and loosely filled with mil-let, can be used to distribute the weight of his skull over a larger area.

When awake, babies lie either on their back, looking at faces and objects and playing with their hands, or on their stomach, which gives them opportunities to hold up their head (and later their shoulders). Babies who usually lie on their back may be a little slower in developing movement, but may have better fine motor skills. If your baby has a definite preference for lying on his back, place him on his stomach for 'tummy time' several times a day while you play and talk with him. If your baby has a hard time falling asleep on his back, try giving him plenty of body contact during the day by carrying him in a sling, and place a rolled-up sweater or other garment belonging to his mother or primary carer in the bed at night.

Always make sure that blankets etc. are placed and secured so that the baby's head cannot possibly slide under them.

12.3 Ways to transport your baby

Many parents find that a sling is their preferred way to carry their child, as long as it is tied correctly and your baby is dressed warmly enough in winter. Slings, like other carrying devices you may use later, allow parents to take their babies with them wherever they go from a very early age. This allows greater mobility and lets the baby experience more of their parents' daily activity. Remember, however, to avoid noisy environments, extreme weather conditions and other sensory impressions that are not appropriate for very young babies (see page 202).

A baby carried by a walking adult experiences rhythmical movement and pressure in their muscles and skin. These sensations not only enhance the baby's sense of self and feeling of comfort but also provide models to imitate in their own later walking, whereas being pushed in a pram is more likely to prepare the baby for driving a car!

When you can no longer avoid using a pram, choose one with a high base and sturdy springs. Large wheels also give a smoother ride. The height protects your baby from car exhaust fumes, which are concentrated near the ground.

If at all possible, try to obtain a pram or stroller in which your baby faces you and can keep eye contact with you. This helps him to learn to observe and focus his attention. Many strollers make the baby face away from the person pushing him, where he is over-whelmed with impressions and is unable to focus or concentrate on anything.

A safe car seat is standard equip-ment. Unfortunately, the design of the safest infant seats supports the baby in an upright position much too early and the resulting 'astronaut posture' constricts the abdomen. If only because car seats restrict movement, infants and toddlers should spend as little time in them as necessary.

12.4 Routine check-ups

Mothers are not always aware that their baby's vital functions are checked immediately after birth. In the UK, this is a legal responsibility for the midwife or paediatrician.

Once you are back home, your local doctor or health visitor will be responsible for following up your baby's progress and giving help and advice with handling and feeding. In some areas, you will be provided with a schedule of rou-tine check-ups for your infant and preschooler. Parents may also be given a record chart or booklet to be kept of the baby's growth and development; in the UK this is called the Personal Child Health Record, referred to informally as the Red Book. This is completed at each check-up and also records the child's immunisations.

The purpose of routine check-ups is to discover, treat and monitor any disturbances or developmental delays, whether physical or psychological, in a timely way. These examinations are a good opportunity for you to keep track of your child's healthy development, since you would otherwise consult a doctor only when your child was ill. The main areas covered in these check-ups are: early recognition of heart defects and congenital hip prob-lems; disorders of development, sensory perception, nutrition and metabolism; prophylactic options including vaccinations and the prevention of rickets and tooth decay; communication disorders and their causes; and questions related to parenting.

Premature infants require spe-cific checks because of the added risks of cerebral palsy or visual problems. Such check-ups and the opportunities they offer for talking with your doctor can help you gain confidence in how your child's development is progressing. The recommended programme for check-ups marks important stages in child development when progress and abilities either become apparent or their absence points to disorders or illness. Because this schedule also coincides with the timing of required or recommended vaccinations, we recommend giving some thought in advance to which optional vaccinations you want your child to receive and which not (see also Chapter 14). Laboratory testing is recommended when a check-up reveals a possible problem. Later check-ups might include urine analysis. At age 4 (or before the child enters kindergarten), a test for tuberculosis may also be performed.

12.5 Breastfeeding

Immediately after birth, the baby is placed on the mother's belly and covered with warmed cloths. Baby, mother and father are given a chance to simply experience each other. If mother and child are both well, the first opportunity to feed follows soon, because babies usually suck forcefully shortly after birth and benefit from receiving the valuable colostrum – the first milk

that breasts produce, which is full of antibodies and immunoglobulins and helps to protect newborns.

Up to the 1970s, for a number of cultural reasons breastfeeding had become quite unusual and even discouraged by modern attitudes. Much has changed in the intervening years. A new culture of breastfeeding has developed, and comprehensive advice is widely available through midwives and La Lèche leaders, who have a wealth of collective experience and literature to answer any detailed questions you may have. Nonetheless, especially among socially disadvantaged populations in many countries, too few mothers today breastfeed their infants. In most Western countries, healthcare services, midwives and breastfeeding counsellors provide recommendations for breastfeeding to every new mother, and we wholeheartedly support this, although we acknowledge that for some mothers and babies breastfeeding is very difficult or even not possible.

Here is a list of reasons for breastfeeding to help mothers everywhere educate themselves and their neighbours about its advantages:
• Breastfeeding creates an intimate bond between a mother and her child and is a very direct way

for both to experience that we humans need each other and are there for each other.

- Mother's milk is always available, sanitary and at the ideal temperature.
- The composition of mother's milk is ideally adapted to the needs of a growing baby.
- In most cases, once mother and baby have mastered the technique, breastfeeding is simple and economical and saves time.
- Breastfeeding stimulates contractions to help shrink the uterus back to its original size after delivery.
- Breastfed babies have fewer and milder infections.
- Breastfeeding largely protects babies against dangerous inflammatory digestive disorders, septicemia and encephalitis.
- Exclusive breastfeeding for the first 6 months may help prevent the development of allergies in the child.

Some practical questions about breastfeeding
How do I learn to breastfeed?

Let your baby teach you! A health visitor, midwife, experienced mother or breastfeeding advisor can also give you tips on different nursing positions, and help with any problems you may encounter.

How often should I breastfeed?

If possible, a mother and her newborn baby should remain together at all times in the first few days after birth. While they are still in the delivery room, babies should be placed on the mother's breast and allowed to nurse as often as they want, even during the night. This means they get all of the highly nourishing colostrum and there is no delay in getting the milk flowing. New mothers should accept offers of competent help and try to relax and get enough sleep between feedings.

Breastfeeding on demand is recommended, which can be as often at 2-hour intervals. At this stage of life a baby belongs at mother's warm breast, hearing her familiar heartbeat. This is especially true of premature infants, who do much better in the 'kangaroo position' than in isolation. We also know that the heartbeats of a mother and her infant tend to become synchronised.

As the baby begins to drink more, the interval between feedings will steadily increase. It is important to learn how to interpret your baby's behaviour. Not every little stretch or sign of discomfort means 'I need to be fed', but if you consistently respond by allowing your baby to nurse, they will make a habit of it and you will not be able to establish a rhythm.

Each feeding should totally empty one breast and at least relieve the pressure on the other.

How long should I breastfeed for?

Most organisations recommend exclusive breastfeeding for at least 6 months, though the World Health Organisation says up to 2 years. Between the ages of 6 and 12 months, most babies gradually wean themselves. Weaning problems are unusual in babies who have had enough physical contact in their first months of life.

What if my breastfed baby doesn't gain weight?

The experienced eye of a health professional is actually just as good as a pair of scales, but if you suspect your baby is not gaining weight rapidly enough, weigh her naked once before a feeding. A second weighing several days later will tell whether she is actually gaining enough weight. **If you are still concerned, seek medical help. Do not delay speaking to your doctor or health visitor with concerns about inadequate weight gain.**

If you need to determine your baby's daily milk consumption, weigh them (in a nappy) before and after each meal for 24 hours: i.e. from the first feeding in the morning to the last one at night. The sum of the differences between weighings is the amount your baby drank that day. By itself, the fact that you may still have milk in your breasts when your baby is finished feeding does not necessarily mean that they aren't getting enough to eat.

What should I eat and drink?

Any normal, healthy foods (preferably organically or biodynamically grown) that are not constipating and do not cause excessive wind. Foods that can make breastfed babies windy include wholegrain bread, raw rolled oats, hot spices, onions and cabbage.

Acceptable beverages include herb teas, low-sodium brands of mineral water, a 7% dilution of almond butter, milk, buttermilk or mild natural yoghurt. Avoid dairy products only if you yourself have eczema related to a milk allergy. If you have symptoms of low blood pressure, drink more fluids and treat yourself to an occasional cup of coffee after feeding. Pressed fruit juices are also acceptable, but don't drink too much at once to begin with. If your baby seems to develop wind or nappy rash when you drink juice, try another kind.

After several weeks, try smaller amounts of the kind that caused the problem.

Can I smoke and breastfeed?

We do not recommend smoking, whether during pregnancy, while breastfeeding or at any other time, not only because of harm to your own health but also harm to your baby's. Smoking during pregnancy significantly reduces birth weight in babies, and smoking while nursing also causes damage because nicotine is excreted in breast milk, not to mention the dangers to your baby of exposure to second-hand smoke. Smoking also increases the risk of sudden infant death (see SIDS, page 214).

Can I drink alcohol and breastfeed?

We recommend complete abstinence from alcohol during pregnancy and breastfeeding. Although it is widely believed that consuming a very small amount of alcohol (no more than 1–2 units once or twice a week) is unlikely to harm your baby, there is still a small risk. Alcohol consumption while breastfeeding may affect your baby's development or cause dependency in the baby that persists even after weaning.

Reasons for not breastfeeding

There are times when a mother might consider not breastfeeding her child for a variety of reasons. We will address some of these below.

What if I don't have enough milk?

Mothers who manage to establish breastfeeding promptly and have enough support from those around them seldom have problems with too little milk. Make sure to drink enough, eat well, get enough rest and keep your upper body and arms (including elbows) warm. It's best to consult a midwife or lactation specialist before resorting to galactagogue teas (made with herbs that increase milk production) or special diets.

We do not recommend giving your baby dairy-based formula in the first few days of life if you intend to breastfeed exclusively later. An allergy-prone baby may become sensitised to cow's milk and develop severe allergic symptoms when she is started on cow's milk for the second time after a long interval of exclusive breastfeeding. There is also a risk that introducing formula makes breastfeeding more difficult in the long run, because your baby will learn to suck at a bottle in a different way to your breast. Giving formula instead of breast milk will probably reduce the amount of breast milk you produce too, because when your baby feeds it sends a signal to your breasts to make more milk. If you do not breastfeed regularly, this signal is not sent and milk production can decrease.

What if breastfeeding is painful?

Although breastfeeding is simple in theory, some women can experience problems with pain for various reasons, some of which we outline below. However, with help, much of the time these can be overcome.

Nipple fissures

These can usually be prevented by ensuring you breastfeed in correct positions, which an experienced midwife or lactation consultant can demonstrate. As preventative skin care for your nipples, allow a little breast milk to dry on them or apply a small amount of St John's wort (Hypericum) oil. Ointments and nipple protectors should be reserved for acute situations.

Milk retention

Even if accompanied by a slight fever, milk retention can be treated with hot, moist (not wet!) compresses or by placing a hot-water bottle on the affected breast 20 minutes before you begin breastfeeding. Massage the breast while your baby is nursing to help press the milk out. Afterward, apply your choice of another hot compress or a cool quark poultice. For deep-seated blockages, eucalyptus paste warmed in a water bath is usually effective. Apply the paste to your breast with a swab.

Mastitis

Mastitis is a condition that causes breasts to become painful and inflamed. Even if accompanied by high fever, it is often possible to continue breastfeeding and it can ease your symptoms. However, treatment by a doctor is necessary.

What if I or my baby are ill?

If you or your baby have an infection or a digestive problem, with or without fever, continue breastfeeding. Your milk will soon change its composition naturally to contain the appropriate antibodies. Unfortunately, gas and abdominal pain are now frequent in breastfed babies (see page 41), so this is not a reason to stop breastfeeding.

What if my breastfed baby has jaundice?

Most newborns, especially breastfed infants, look a bit yellow for

Milk donation

If you have more than enough milk, consider donating the excess to a milk bank so it can be given to a baby who needs it. Many premature and critically ill infants owe their lives to this kind of help. Ask your doctor or health visitor about your nearest milk bank and how to make donations. The process is rigorous and the milk bank will send you a questionnaire and a blood-testing kit, to test for illnesses such as HIV, syphilis and hepatitis. (Make an appointment with your doctor or a nurse to take the bloods.) If you are accepted by the milk bank after your blood has been tested, you will be sent instructions on how to store your milk hygienically and bottles in which to freeze it before it is picked up.

several days or weeks after delivery. This condition is generally harmless. For severe jaundice, see page 95.

What if I have a serious illness or long-term health condition?

Consult your doctor for advice. As examples, mothers with active tuberculosis or (in some cases) an advanced milk gland abscess should not breastfeed. Breastfeeding if you have HIV depends on the stage of the infection and requires consulting a specialist.

What if I am taking medication?

Whenever your doctor prescribes a medication for you, ask whether it might harm your nursing infant and (if possible) choose a medication that is not excreted in breast milk.

After dental work involving local anaesthesia, pump out your milk once or twice and throw it away, to ensure the anaesthesia has left your milk before you resume breastfeeding your baby. If you have plenty of milk, you can pump before your dental work and refrigerate it in a sterile bottle in anticipation of this time when you should not breastfeed.

12.6 Bottle-feeding

It is extremely important that babies get enough milk, in order to stay hydrated and grow and develop well. **It is vital to seek medical help if you are worried that your baby is not drinking enough milk, is not passing stools, has a dry nappy or is not gaining weight.** If assistance with breastfeeding does not produce the desired results, or if you and your doctor or midwife agree your baby needs feed supplements for any reason – which often happens – there are a range of options available. You can express your own breast milk and spoon or bottle-feed it to your baby. You can use milk donated from another mother by contacting a milk bank (see above). You may be able to find a doctor, midwife or breastfeeding consultant who has experience with natural, dairy-based supplemental formulas. For further advice we would recommend contacting La Lèche League (see Further Resources, page 319).

Commercial formulas are widely used and available; they are easy to handle and most babies digest them well. A quick look at the composition of formulas reveals very careful attempts to adjust their ingredients to correspond to the nutritional value of breast milk. In addition to adequate amounts of all imaginable trace elements, minerals, and vitamins, every formula includes a few chemicals that make the product economically competitive by improving its appearance, shelf life and taste. It seems clear to us, however, that all these ingredients do not add up to a living, whole food. The fact that most food allergies appeared only after the invention of formula is also food for thought.

How to bottle-feed your baby
You can still nourish your baby

Formula feeding tips

- Babies' immune systems are still developing, so they are susceptible to illness and infection. It is vital to sterilise babies' feeding equipment until they are at least 1 year old.
- After sterilising, leave bottles and teats in the steriliser or pan of water until you need them.
- Wash and dry your hands before handling sterile feeding equipment, or use sterile tongs.
- Follow the manufacturer's instructions carefully; different formulas use different amounts of water and powder.
- Do not use water that has been boiled before.
- Do not use bottled water to make up feeds, as it may contain too much salt or sulphate.
- Do not add extra formula powder, because this can make your baby constipated or dehydrated.
- Do not heat up formula in a microwave as it can create 'hot spots' and burn your baby's mouth.
- Make up feeds one at a time as you need them.
- Throw away any formula left after a feed.

---

well and feel a close bond with your baby during the process of bottle-feeding. Hold your baby upright, support his head and look into his eyes. When the formula has cooled enough to drink, brush the teat against your baby's lips and allow him to draw the teat into his mouth. Angle the bottle so that the teat is constantly full of milk; otherwise your baby may take in too much air and get windy (see below for advice on burping your baby). Stay with your baby while he is feeding from a bottle and never allow him to feed alone from a propped-up bottle. If you need more guidance, ask your doctor or health visitor.

12.7 Excretions and other bodily functions

Burping a baby after drinking

All babies swallow a certain amount of air while drinking, especially if they are bottle-fed. To minimise possetting (spitting up) and to allow your baby to sleep as comfortably as possible, the resulting air bubble in the stomach needs to be released upward. This is done by holding your baby with his chin resting on your shoulder, which you should cover with a cloth to catch any milk that's brought up. Unfortunately, many parents then proceed to clap their baby quickly and repeatedly on the back. It is much more comfortable

for the baby if you sit down with them leaning against you and stroke their head very gently.

Hiccups

Hiccups are caused by spasmodic, rhythmical contractions of the diaphragm. Hiccups are easily triggered by a cold draught on the baby's stomach, by putting the baby down or turning them over too quickly, or by a strong burp. Often, however, they occur for no apparent reason. In newborns, hiccups mean that parents will wait in vain for a burp but can be sure that the baby will not posset (spit up), simply because the diaphragm's contractions temporarily keep the entrance to the stomach closed. Placing a warm cloth on the baby's abdomen can help to prevent hiccups.

Consistency and frequency of stools

After discharge of the black or dark green meconium, which accumulates in the bowel of the foetus in the last few weeks of pregnancy, a breastfed infant's stools are yellow or light green with very mild odour. Occasionally they may be very fluid, dark yellow and contain only lentil-shaped solid particles of a cheesy consistency.

Frequency generally varies between 2 and 6 times a day,

but breastfed babies' bowel movements can be as frequent as 10 times a day or as infrequent as once every 10 days. This is no cause for alarm as long as the baby has no other symptoms and seems to be thriving.

The stools usually change when other foods are introduced. The smell becomes less pleasant, the colour yellow or brownish, the consistency mushy or paste-like, the frequency generally 2–4 times a day but at least every other day. At this point, a yeasty smell is a possible sign of a fungal infection (Candida albicans), while a green colour and loose stools indicate a mild digestive disturbance (dyspepsia).

Consult your doctor immediately if your infant's stools contain traces of blood, including threads of haematin blackened by contact with stomach acid (not to be confused with banana fibres, which look similar!) or if they are bleached, greyish-white, and accompanied by obvious jaundice.

Urination

In the first few months of life, an infant's urine is almost colourless; it becomes somewhat more yellow only in cases of pronounced jaundice. Urine left in nappies for some time develops a biting odour of ammonia, especially if the baby is formula-fed. Ammonia exacerbates nappy rash, so if you notice this odour, change your baby's nappies more frequently and pay special attention to skincare and cleaning (with water only). If the weather is hot and your baby has not been drinking much, her urine can easily develop a reddish-orange colour due to precipitation of harmless phosphate salts. To rectify this, ensure your baby drinks more.

Painful urination is often due to a urinary tract infection; in such cases the urine usually smells bad or at least markedly different than usual. Urinary tract infections should be diagnosed and treated by a physician. **If 2 meals pass without a wet nappy, your baby may be feverish or dehydrated; other symptoms will determine whether professional advice is needed. Always consult your doctor if you are concerned.**

Perspiration

Perspiration is unusual in the first few months of life, but it can occur if the baby is overheated, drinks a great deal or has a fever. It may also be due to vegetative disorders that usually cannot be pinned down. Increased perspiration for no apparent reason when your baby is around 6 weeks old may be a sign of early-stage rickets (see page 255). Consult your doctor about rickets prevention.

12.8 Nappy (diaper) changing and washing your baby

The vernix caseosa – the white creamy substance that covers the newborn baby's skin at birth — is a natural protection absorbed by the skin after a few hours. Bathing is unnecessary immediately after birth; traces of blood can usually be dabbed off with a cloth.

Choosing nappies (diapers)

Increasingly, parents are avoiding disposable nappies for newborn babies because cloth nappies keep babies warmer and save on waste disposal. Newborn babies can wear gauze nappies covered with soakers (woollen pants) or the like (see page 315). After changing, wrap your baby in a large brushed cotton or flannel cloth (wool is also very practical for this purpose) instead of rompers or leggings. Depending on the season, you may need to add a loosely knitted wool blanket over everything.

Babies born in the breech position often have immature hip joints and need wide nappies from the very beginning to hold their legs apart. An extra cotton cloth folded into a broad strip and placed between the legs usually does the trick.

When your baby begins to kick his way out of his swaddling (usually after a few weeks), onesies or babygrows with snaps between the legs are a practical solution. At this point, you will probably find that it works well to combine 2 gauze nappies: a triangular one for wrapping and a rectangular one placed between the baby's legs. A little later, you may want to add a nappy liner for easier clean-up. Soakers made of unbleached wool hold everything in place. Add wool rompers for daytime wear. At night, cotton rompers may be more practical; on top, wrap your baby in the knitted wool blanket mentioned above so that they are not always kicking freely, but can feel some resistance, thus sensing themselves.

We do not recommend allowing your baby complete freedom of movement all the time from a very early age. If you observe your baby's many involuntary and reflexive movements during the first few months of life, you will notice that they interfere with the baby's ability to look around. The need to support the activity of quiet looking is evident when you realise that the calmer and more alert a baby's gaze, the more readily they learn to use their hands. Hence it is important to choose a nappy technique that puts the brakes on extensive kicking gestures and limits your baby's movements.

Do not wrap your baby so tightly, however, that the hip joints have no freedom of movement at all. Too tight nappies can have negative effects on the development of the hip joint sockets, a special consideration in cases of hip dysplasia (underdeveloped hip sockets) or weak ligaments that cause loose hip joints. In these cases, the hip may eventually dislocate. It is important to recognise and treat hip problems as early as possible. If you are concerned about this, a diagnosis can be confirmed through ultrasound imaging. If hip dysplasia or congenital dislocation of the hip are overlooked and are noticed only because of the baby's wobbly gait when they learn to walk, surgical correction (usually involving several operations) becomes necessary.

If you carry your baby in a sling from the very beginning, first lay them diagonally on a wool blanket, turning the lower corner up over the legs and wrapping the side corners around the baby so that their whole body, including the feet, is already warmly enclosed when you put them into the sling.

Washing, bathing and skincare

An infant's skin, like that of adults, has a fine layer of natural oils whose quality cannot be duplicated. It makes no sense to wash these oils off every day and replace them with other fats. In most cases, one bath a week is enough for infants. Between baths, wash your baby's face, nappy area and the folds of their skin daily with a soft washcloth and comfortably warm water (no soap). Cleaning with plain water without soap is usually enough even for areas soiled by urine, stools or vomit. Stuck remnants of stools or nappy rash ointments are fat-soluble and can be removed with sunflower seed oil, which is more economical for cleaning than skincare oils.

The best baby oils for skincare contain calendula or chamomile oil. Apply a thin layer of one of these oils to the folds of skin on your baby's neck, under the arms, behind the ears and in the nappy area.

Do not use powder on these areas because it can combine

with moisture and become crumbly, causing irritation. In any case, clouds of powder can make your baby cough and are dangerous for her lungs.

Fun on the changing table

In early infancy, a considerable part of a baby's contact with their parents takes place on the changing table. At changing time, infants are generally well fed, in a good mood, and ready to enjoy movement and contact. The minutes during and after cleaning, washing and oiling your baby's skin can serve both necessary and playful purposes. Hum, sing and talk with your child and play with their hands and feet. After a few weeks, you can expect to hear their first contact-seeking sounds in response. As the months go by, playtime on the changing table can become increasingly lively as your baby begins to ask to be picked up and learns to turn over and then to crawl. At that point, you need to keep your wits about you to make sure that your baby has something interesting in their hands to keep them occupied so they won't fall off the table. If your baby is really lively, it may be safer to change them on the floor.

With the exception of medically prescribed massage, we advise against regular, systematic massages for infants, although they are currently very popular and recommended with enthusiasm. For infants, physical attention should arise spontaneously out of natural needs and should not be programmed. Your infant's need for deep pressure sensations (which make him feel comfortable in his surroundings) is naturally met by being carried on your arm or in a sling (see also page 188). Their own desire to move and explore will provide all the other tactile sensations they need.

This process of discovery is two-sided. Every time your baby looks at or touches something, pulls himself upright or crawls, he is learning to 'grasp' both his surroundings and himself. Everything adults do with infants includes an additional factor – the attitude with which the action is performed. Anxious holding back, effusive exaggeration, hectic activity, consciously or unconsciously applied educational principles, fear of spoiling the baby, the desire to ensure that your baby is physically fit: we recommend making the effort to check these behaviours so that you can respond appropriately to your baby's advances. Patience and a cheerful, loving attitude, not anxieties and specific ideas about what to do, will help you provide imaginative, spontaneous, and helpful stimuli.

12.9 Cultivating early sense impressions

Sounds and tones

Even if the baby makes no sound, our behaviour changes instinctively and immediately when we enter a newborn's room. Even lively and rumbunctious children quietly approach the cradle on tiptoe. Conversely, everyone around the new baby come running when they scream. The parents' words and expressions of pleasure and loving attention interact subtly with every sound the baby utters.

Even before birth, a baby's sense of hearing is fully functional and their body is profoundly affected by voices and noises in their parents' surroundings. We recommend exposing unborn and newborn babies to as little recorded music and mechanical noise as possible. Everything we do with children in their first few years of life has profound effects on their development and contributes to habits that may persist for the rest of their lives.

Initially, any mechanical noise – whether from construction equipment outside or vacuum cleaners and dishwashers inside – is foreign and disturbing. Sleeping babies often react to this type of noise with a change in breathing or a faster pulse. We adults need to consider whether the sounds in a baby's environment are age-appropriate. Our auditory experience occupies a spectrum ranging from absolute silence through a multitude of human, instrumental and mechanical sounds. The more sensitive and careful you are about your baby's auditory environment, the subtler the sounds they will later be able to distinguish.

As paediatricians, we often have to ask mothers who phone us about their feverish infants to turn off the radio blaring in the background. Before children learn to speak and think, they have no way of preserving any distance between themselves and the impressions – especially noises – that their surroundings impose on them. The ability to distance oneself from perceptions develops only gradually, as a result of naming things and thinking about them.

In the first year of life especially, a child is totally incapable of shutting out the external world; the child's entire body is highly sensitive and is forced to participate in all the impressions that affect it.

Subtle or not-so-subtle changes in respiratory and circulatory rhythms are a sensitive indicator of these impacts. Of course this does not mean that we need to refrain from all enjoyment of music when there is a baby in the house, but it does mean that we should attempt to keep it at some distance from the baby and to adapt our selections to their sensitivity.

As much as possible, babies should be spared mechanical noises and 'acoustic bombardment' with media such as radio, television, videos and recorded music.

The powerful effects of sounds and tones on infants are evident when we watch them play. If you put a plastic rattle in your baby's hand or suspend a noise-producing mobile over their cradle, the effect is clear from the baby's movements. It is as if their kicking gestures are directed inward, shaking their body. The effect of playing with a simple wooden clapper with its sliding part is totally different. The baby's movements adapt to the sounds they perceive and become noticeably more deliberate and regular. In both cases, the baby seems happy and excited by the noise, but in the latter instance, they seem more composed, self-contained and able to process the sense impression.

Still different is the impact of a simple series of notes sung or hummed by the parent. The baby pauses in amazement, their movements become more relaxed and, if they are tired, they soon fall asleep. When the baby opens themselves up to these tones, they become more able to surrender their soul to sleep.

Fresh air and humidity

Everyone agrees that infants need fresh air, but when we open a window in a big city, we have to take what we can get. Exposing your baby to cool air is fine, but do avoid draughts – another practical reason for a veil over the child's bed (see page 186). Whether or not and for how long to open a window depends not only on the outdoor temperature and noise but also on indoor dryness. A good solution is to open the window wide several times a day when the baby is in another room. Avoid exposing your baby to cooking odours or cigarette smoke, however.

With regard to moisture in the air, most modern heating systems dry out the air and are unsuitable for children. Water containers suspended from the radiators help but do not evaporate enough water (several litres/quarts a day) to totally replace lost moisture. This level of humidification can be achieved only with electrical devices, which you may not want to use for other reasons (noise, bacterial risks and so on). If you must purchase a humidifier for health reasons, such as frequent colds in the family, make sure to get one that operates without a motor, uses ordinary tap water and does not require a filter. This type of humidifier brings water to the boiling point between two electrode plates.

If you do not have a humidifier, the best alternative is to air the baby's room briefly but frequently. Alternatively, you can keep water steaming on a small electric hot-plate (out of children's reach!) set on low. When your baby has a respiratory infection, adding a few drops of pure eucalyptus oil to this water (not directly on to the heater) enhances the quality of the humidified air and reduces the effects of irritants such as ozone and nitrogen oxide.

Sunlight

In semi-darkness, newborn babies open their eyes and seem to be looking for something, but if you let light fall directly into the cradle, their eyes close again immediately. After a few weeks, however, they begin to look around in different directions even when the room is brighter. Now is the time to let your baby sleep by an open window or outside, protected from wind and direct sun. It is important to expose your baby's face to the blue sky (see Rickets, page 255). Begin with 15 minutes to half an hour a day, depending on the weather, and gradually increase to 2 hours or longer. Of course you'll need to check on your baby occasionally, even if they are sleeping.

The mere thought of putting a 3- or 4-week-old infant to bed outside under a clear blue sky is abhorrent to some people, even if the baby is warmly covered and wearing a cap, but in temperate latitudes this is one of the best steps you can take to ensure your baby's healthy physical development. Next to mother's milk, light from a clear blue sky is the most effective way to stimulate healthy bone growth.* An infant whose

---

* The ultraviolet radiation wavelengths that prevent rickets are transmitted much better through blue sky overhead than through the paler sky near the horizon. We believe that the polarisation of sunlight is also important. It enables bees to orient themselves in space, and with a little practise humans can also perceive Haidinger's brushes (a fleeting pale yellow image like a stack of hay). The structure of the sky as a whole in relationship to the sun certainly has very different effects from a plain blue, radiant surface.

forehead is exposed to blue sky for 2 hours a day will not develop rickets.

In cloudy climates or industrial areas where blue sky may not be seen for months on end, other steps must be taken to prevent rickets, but they are usually not necessary in areas with more sun. We urgently advise you not to expose your child to too much light early in life – no sunbathing that exposes all or most of their skin, for example. Too much light causes premature hardening throughout the body and overtaxes the nervous system. To confirm this statement, simply consider the state of your own skin and mental acuity after excessive sunbathing. Here, too, moderation is in order.

Heat and cold

A newborn baby's thermoregulatory system is immature and easily disrupted (see Rhythms, page 244). Infants delivered in cold surroundings tend to have subnormal body temperatures for hours afterwards, even if they are wrapped warmly right after birth. Doctors and parents are still learning how important it is to keep babies consistently warm during the first few days and weeks of life.

Whatever the situation, make sure that your baby does not get cold. For example, a fan heater in the bathroom is not as good as a radiant heater, but the radiant heater should also not be located directly over the baby's head. Marbled skin colouration or a red, hot head will let you know you've made a mistake. Outdoors, cool cheeks and cool exposed hands are normal in warmly dressed babies. Under a blanket, however, hands and feet should always be comfortably warm. A baby's uncovered head radiates a lot of heat and should therefore be covered with a woollen cap outside and a light one, perhaps of cotton or silk, inside. Hot days and hot climates are exceptions to this rule, but in these situations your baby should wear a sunhat.

In the first few weeks of your baby's life, you may need to place a warmed sack of cherrystones or grains in their bed for extra warmth (do not use a hot-water bottle because of the danger of leaking and scalding). Be careful not to make it too hot, though! Even 40°C/104°F can 'burn' a baby's sensitive skin after a while. If your baby's room is cool or if you prefer not to use a featherbed, cover your baby with a woollen sleeping bag or a blanket of similar weight.

If your baby often has cool hands for no apparent reason, it usually helps to dress them in a long-sleeved woollen undershirt. Try to find a brand of wool under-wear that is soft enough for your baby, but if you can't find wool of this quality, use a thin cotton undershirt under woollen cloth-ing. We also recommend woollen nappy covers and rompers because wool has the unique ability to absorb up to 30% of its own weight in water without feeling damp and can evaporate moisture without cooling the skin. Wool also draws away perspiration better than any synthetic fibre and is less likely to trap heat next to the skin. This is why desert Bedouin wear clothing made of wool or sheepskins.

Some people object to wool because it feels scratchy against their skin. Even soft wool becomes scratchy if it mats or felts, so wash your baby's wool garments carefully in lukewarm water and a suitable detergent. Undershirts and bonnets of raw silk are good for babies with very sensitive skin. This fabric regu-lates warmth nearly as well as wool and is extremely comfortable to wear. Generally, pure cotton under-wear by itself is practical only when the weather is very warm and tem-peratures do not fluctuate much, or where your baby has a wool and silk allergy. Synthetics are to be avoided, because they trap body heat and do not absorb moisture.

We have discussed wool clothing in such detail because as paediatricians we all too fre-quently see infants who are not dressed warmly enough. We only rarely see the other extreme – a baby dressed in layer upon layer of wool, with a wool cap coming right down to her eyebrows so that even her forehead is not allowed to be cool. Seeing these two extremes of excessive cooling and excessive warmth makes it easy to under-stand the need for moderation – everything at the right time and in the right place. Too much warmth overprotects the body and pre-vents it from developing effective internal thermoregulation. And at this stage of life, too little warmth – or worse still, deliberate exposure to cold – establishes reflexes that bear no relationship to normal cir-cumstances and therefore trigger excessive reactions. In either case, the baby cannot learn to respond flexibly and moderately to changes in temperature.

12.10 Spontaneous movement development

The motto 'all education is self-ed-ucation' certainly applies to learn-ing to move. We adults often need to learn that babies naturally want to imitate and explore. Allowing your baby to discover all the new and different possibilities of human movement for themselves takes much patience and willingness to simply observe. It is important to arrange your baby's surroundings in ways that allow them to explore it for themselves, along with ever-new opportunities to learn and master the laws of movement and balance. Independence in learning how to move not only ensures balanced and lasting bodily stability but also helps babies learn to trust their own possibilities and gain a sense of autonomy and 'freedom'.

It hardly needs to be mentioned that each baby has their own 'schedule' of motor development. Your child will benefit if you wait patiently for each new movement pattern to emerge (turning over, wriggling forward on their elbows, crawling, pulling themselves upright, walking with and without support) and refrain from providing permanent supports or a 'helping hand'. Learning these movements on their own provides a lifelong basis for development in other areas.

Swimming for infants

With few exceptions, we do not recommend swimming or outdoor bathing for infants. These activities are usually associated with temperature fluctuations, chlorine or pollutants in the water, and other children's yelling, all of which can overtax a baby's highly sensitive system.

Your infant's motor development will be quite adequately stimulated by spontaneous movement, the joy of repetition and little games with adults who take pride in each new movement they master. It is important, however, to find time for such games and activities on a daily basis. Sitting in front of the television with the baby in your arms does not count!

12.11 Common conditions in newborn babies

Broken collarbone

This relatively common birth injury may be missed when the doctor examines your child after delivery; later, however, swelling around the break makes it obvious. This type of fracture always heals without intervention, and symptoms disappear after a few days.

Symptoms

- Pain when your baby is dressed, laid down or when their shoulders are moved.
- Possible ridge or swelling can be felt around the collarbone.

How you can help

- Take care when dressing babies and laying them down.
- To avoid a skull deformity, be careful to alternate head positions when you lay your baby down (see page 187).

Remedies

- Arnica planta tota Rh 3X, 5 drops 3–6 times daily – keep drops refrigerated.
- Symphytum comp. glob. velati, 3 globules 3 times a day.

Wryneck (muscular torticollis)

This is caused by slight rupturing of the muscle during delivery. Untreated, this condition causes deformation of the head (see page 187).

Symptoms

- Infant always holds the head tilted to one side with the chin pointing slightly in the other direction.
- Slight swelling in the sterno-cleidomastoid muscle (between breastbone and collarbone) on the side in question.
- Excessive stretching of the muscle causes pain.

How you can help

- A program of careful stretching, implemented by a doctor or physical therapist, usually restores the balance.
- Arnica ointment, once or twice a day.

Pyloric stenosis in the first 3 months

Pyloric stenosis is a condition in which food is blocked from entering the small intestine. A doctor should examine your baby if they stop gaining or lose weight. Some children may need medication or perhaps even surgery (fortunately, the operation is not very invasive).

Symptoms

- Appears most commonly between the second and fourth week of life.
- Projectile vomiting.
- Symptoms tend to increase over several days.
- Weight loss may occur in severe cases.
- No diarrhoea or fever.

How you can help

- Check your baby's weight 2–3 times a week.
- Give more frequent, smaller meals.
- Mothers should try to get as much quiet and peace as possible.
- Take your time burping your baby.
- Apply a warm abdominal

compress made with cham-omile tea, lemon balm tea or oxalis essence (see page 305).

- Apply a warmed cherry-stone pillow on your baby's abdomen.

Remedies

- Gently rub your baby's lower abdomen with copper ointment.
- Chamomilla Cupro culta, Radix Rh 3X, 5 drops before each meal.

Gastro-oesophageal reflux in the first 3 months

Gastro-oesophageal reflux occurs when the valve at the entrance to the stomach does not close completely, allowing peristaltic movements of the stomach to force food back up into your baby's oesophagus. The stomach valve usually matures in a few weeks or months.

Brownish threads of blood in the vomit should be reported to your doctor immediately, because they indicate that gastric juices are damaging the oesophagus. However, medication to reduce the acidity of the stomach or surgery is seldom necessary.

Symptoms

- Frequent dribbly vomiting or possetting (spitting up) in a broad stream in the first few weeks of life.
- Possetting (spitting up) while nursing, while burping or when lying down.

How you can help

- Allow plenty of time while feed-ing, feeding for short spells and lifting your baby in between.
- Take plenty of time burping your baby.
- Your doctor may advise you to raise the head of your baby's cradle or crib so that she lies on an incline (of about 30°) with her head higher than her legs. **Ensure that your baby cannot slip under their blanket.**

Remedies

- Before each meal Chamomilla Cupro culta, Radix Rh 3X, 5 drops OR
- Nicotiana comp. glob. velati, 3 globules.
- Stronger remedies that reduce the acidity of the gastric juices are rarely necessary.

12.12 Skin conditions in babies

Acne

Almost all babies develop a non-itching rash usually starting on the back and the face. It is quite harmless and has nothing to do with allergies or neurodermatitis. However, some newborns are now developing eczema so early that it is difficult to distinguish it from neonatal acne or other postnatal rashes, and is only later recognised as a problem in its own right.

Causes
- Hormonal adjustment after birth

Symptoms
- Rash with non-itching little pimples
- In pronounced cases, suppurative pimples
- Usually begins in the face, infrequently on the back
- Location frequently changes during progression
- Lasts up to 3 months

How you can help
- Avoid creams and lotions.
- Occasionally wash or bathe the affected areas with thyme tea.

Rashes
Causes
- Hormonal adjustment after birth

Symptoms
- Irregularly distributed, yellowish, pinhead-sized nodules surrounded by relatively large, irregularly bounded reddened areas.
- Location frequently changes.

How you can help
- Avoid creams and lotions.

- Rash disappears on its own within a few days.

Milia (whiteheads)
Milia (whiteheads) are caused by retention of keratin in oil gland ducts. In the mouth, Epstein pearls (on the gums or at the junction of the hard and soft palates) are sometimes confused with thrush (see page 100).

Symptoms
- Firm, white pimples the size of pinheads on a newborn baby's skin.
- Usually around the eyes.
- In the mouth, somewhat larger spots (Epstein pearls) on the gums or at the junction of the hard and soft palates.

How you can help
- Whiteheads usually disappear by themselves.
- Later occurrences, which can be more persistent, can be washed with sage tea.

Pimples on the cheeks
Pimples on the cheeks in the first few weeks of a baby's life are, like adolescent acne, due to hormonal changes. However, pimples in infants are filled with sebum rather than pus; they are not contagious and are a common manifestation of seborrhoeic

dermatitis (see page 114). They should be distinguished from pimples filled with pus that appear later in childhood (see page 116, Eczema).

Symptoms
• Rough pimples on the cheeks

How you can help
• Use a mild skincare cream from your pharmacy, i.e. almond oil creams.

Pustules and blisters

In contrast to the generally pointed, firm and yellowish nodules of a seborrhoeic skin rash on the cheeks, pustules or blisters are somewhat flat, usually a few millimeters in diameter and greenish yellow in colour contain actual pus and are a suppurative skin condition. The pus contains colonies of staphylococcus (staph) bacteria. We are dealing with this here, because in infants it looks different and needs to be treated differently.

Staph infections not only appear when hygiene is inadequate, but also in families who overuse antiseptics. These destroy the normal skin flora, resulting in increased susceptibility to colonisation by germs.

It is important to know that these infections can be easily transmitted to other young infants whose immune systems are still immature. Nursing mothers may also get a breast infection.

Symptoms
• Somewhat flat greenish-yellow pustules or blisters, usually a few millimeters in diameter.
• The pustules occur either singly or in groups and usually appear on the skin of the head, armpits or nappy area, although they may also appear anywhere else on the body.
• In infrequent cases, pus-filled blisters 1 centimeter or more (½ in) in diameter can develop in a matter of hours.

How you can help
• Change your baby's clothes and sheets completely once a day, as well as all bath and hand towels.
• Squeeze ointments onto disposable applicators instead of your fingers.
• Clean out the bag that holds your babycare supplies. You may need to throw out the supplies and buy new ones.
• Thoroughly wash your hands with soap and scrub with a fingernail brush before and after washing your baby.
• Keep your fingernails short to minimise harbouring of germs.

- Avoid letting your hair touch your infant, because it can harbour bacteria.
- Do whatever you can to minimise the spread of germs.
- Seek medical care, especially if fever develops or if symptoms develop very quickly.
- Under medical supervision, staph infections can usually be treated with thyme tea. Occasionally a topical cream containing fusidic acid, and in severe cases antibiotics (orally or as infusion), are needed.
- As a supporting measure give Calendula 4X glob. 3–5 globules 4 times daily.

Yellow skin colouration (jaundice)
- See page 95.

Inflamed navel
Symptoms
- Moist, reddened navel that might even bleed slightly after the second week post-birth.
- Little pimples around the navel.
- If severely inflamed, red and swollen skin.

How you can help
- If mildly irritated or moist, dab the navel with sage tincture.
- In more severe cases, apply powder (Wecesin, for example) and see your doctor.

Umbilical granuloma
Symptoms
- Pea-sized inflammation ('proud flesh') at the spot where the umbilical cord was attached.
- Possible slight bleeding.

How you can help
- Go to your doctor, who will simply dab the spot with a silver nitrate 'pencil'.
- If the navel remains moist, try dabbing the navel with sage tincture.

Nappy (diaper) rash
In common parlance, 'nappy rash' means any and all inflammatory skin symptoms in the nappy area.

Causes
- Leaving stools in the nappy for too long.
- Unusually irritating stools, for example, after giving your baby orange juice or apples.
- Mild digestive disturbances (more frequent during teething).
- Beginnings of diarrhoea.

Symptoms
- Sudden, bright redness of the skin around the anus, usually not extending beyond the folds in the buttocks.

How you can help
- Clean the rash first with water,

then with almond or olive oil.
- Dry the area thoroughly and apply a fat-based ointment that adheres well (e.g. zinc oxide ointment with cod-liver oil or Weleda baby cream).
- Change nappies frequently.

Thrush
Symptoms
- Little red pimples with thin rings of white scales around the edges.
- First appears around the anus or genitals, possibly merging and spreading to cover the entire nappy area all the way to the navel.
- Uniformly red, firm surface that tends to ooze.

How you can help
- See page 100.

Seborrhoeic dermatitis
Symptoms
- Yellowy, scaly inflammation of the skin.

How you can help
- See page 114.

Ammonia dermatitis
Causes
- Nappies are not changed often enough.
- Overly rough cleaning of these sensitive areas.

Chafing nappies or plastic pants
Symptoms
- Skin irritation in the folds of the groin or around the stomach.

How you can help
- Dab the area clean with generous amounts of oil.
- Treat the patches with a fat-based, additive-free cream or ointment.
- Don't use powder, because it can form crumbs and cause further irritation. Powder can also cause your baby to cough or even choke.

Suitable detergents
During the first few weeks of a baby's life, a relatively dense rash of pimples or blisters may appear, extending beyond the nappy area to the upper body. Such rashes are not always clearly either bacterial or fungal in origin.

Experience shows that they disappear quickly if you simply eliminate fabric softeners and give each washload an extra rinse, perhaps adding a little vinegar. For cotton fabrics in direct contact with the skin, use a dryer, which makes the fibres softer. Avoiding the use of fabric softeners and using unscented detergents has proven especially helpful in cases of sensitive or allergic skin.

12.13 Sudden infant death syndrome (SIDS)

Sudden infant death syndrome, otherwise known as 'cot death', is listed as the cause of ⅓ of all fatalities between the end of the first month and the end of the first year of life. In the majority of cases, the children are discovered lifeless in their beds.

Possible causes

Recent studies in many different countries reveal a series of statistical factors that increase the risk of sudden infant death:

- Cramped living quarters
- Adults who smoke during pregnancy and after delivery
- Premature babies (before 33rd week)
- Siblings who died of SIDS
- Allowing the babies to sleep on their stomach or side (see also page 187)
- Allowing babies to sleep in their parents' bed (especially if they smoke)
- Putting babies to bed in an overheated room or under over-insulating covers, or dressing them in a warm cap or bonnet for sleeping
- Covers that the baby can slide under
- Excessive cooling
- Formula feeding rather than breastfeeding

- Previous acute life-threatening event, or ALTE. This is the term applied to a case where the infant survives, either through resuscitation or because they begin breathing again on their own.

How you can help

- Avoid the possible causes listed above.
- If there is a high risk, take extra care. Consider using a baby monitor.
- Immediately begin resuscitation if you find your infant lifeless (see page 13).

Assuming that certain infants are predisposed to SIDS as a result of seizure disorders or disturbances in respiratory regulation, specialised laboratory equipment has been developed to simultaneously monitor heart rhythm, respiration rate, brain waves, blood gas levels and other factors on a 24-hour basis (called polysomnography). When excessively long pauses in respiration are suspected in an infant, electronic monitoring of respiration in the hospital for several days can help to assess the risk of SIDS. Today, these tests are performed on all infants who are either medically at risk or who have survived an ALTE.

It is important to realise, however, that only 10–25% of SIDS cases occur in children considered medically at risk. This means that there is little overlap between tested children and those truly at risk. Cases of SIDS have been known to occur even when polysomnograms (with or without subsequent consistent monitoring) revealed no cause for alarm.

Simply educating the public about the risk of allowing babies to sleep on their stomachs has led to an almost 50% reduction of SIDS cases in some areas. The low rate of SIDS in the Netherlands is attributed to the practice of putting babies to bed on their backs in sleeping bags that extend up to the armpits; this practice has now become widespread in other parts of the world too. For practical details about sleeping positions, see page 187.

Other statistical studies, which found pertussis germs in some autopsied infants, conclude that early, undiagnosed stages of whooping cough contribute to some cases of sudden infant death (see Section 7.9).

Thoughts on dealing with sudden death

One mother whose infant son survived an ALTE wrote us this letter:

The survival of our 2-month-old son raised many questions in us, as parents, about his destiny and path in life. There is no satisfactory medical explanation for this phenomenon; we must look for answers in other domains. It has become increasingly clear to us that our son's near-death experience and return to his body will probably influence his entire life. He has changed in positive ways since this event. The alertness, clarity and radiance of his facial expression give the impression of someone who has been born a second time. Our concern about our child has disappeared gradually, replaced by a sense of security provided by electronic monitoring.

This boy's mother found him lying lifeless in bed and was unable to resuscitate him herself, but he was revived in the ambulance on the way to the hospital and released after 2 weeks in intensive care and in the paediatric ward. His condition was monitored electronically after the event. This is one of the rare cases where an infant was resuscitated after being found in a lifeless state.

Parents who lose a child to SIDS face questions that we believe can only be explored on a spiritual level. Why did their child leave their body?

A riddle confronts anyone familiar with the will to live displayed by infants and premature babies and the difficulties they have to overcome. Was this merely an attempt at incarnation? Was a fresh start required because it became apparent that the body that had developed thus far was actually unsuited to the earthly life the individual had planned?

Some mothers who lose a child to SIDS and soon become pregnant again have the strong impression that it is the same child, while others do not.

We are still extremely ignorant about the possibilities of life before birth (see also Section 15). Are SIDS children trying to alert us to the threshold to the spiritual worlds, where birth and death hold out their hands to each other?

These children leave behind questions directed to us, to the earthly world and especially to the world where the dead and the not-yet-born meet. As we work on these questions, our life is deepened and enriched: another reason for being grateful for the gift of the short time these children spend with us.

12.14 Introducing solid foods

Nutrition and allergy experts now recommend this basic approach:
- Breast milk is the optimal exclusive food for babies under 6 months.
- **If possible, delay introducing cow's milk and other dairy products. Cow's milk should not be given as your baby's main drink before the age of 1.**
- Instead, beginning at 6 months, gradually introduce a variety of supplemental foods including vegetables, fruit and grains.

After the age of 6 months, gradually increasing amounts of vegetables, fruit or cereals can be offered after a milk meal. Introduce no more than one new food per week. Try giving your baby apples (either cooked or raw and grated); cooked pears, peaches, plums, or cherries; or pureed berries (either straight or added to cereals). As soon as your baby tolerates a steamed fruit or vegetable, you can also give her a raw piece to gnaw on, which provides new opportunities for touching, biting, tasting and swallowing. These experiences encourage your child's initiative and independence with regard to foods.

Vegetables should be steamed and enriched with a teaspoon of good-quality vegetable oil. Nitrate-rich vegetables such as carrots, beetroot and spinach should not be a frequent choice. Use them as fresh as possible, and do not reheat vegetables of this type for your baby's use.

Gluten-free grains (rice, buckwheat corn, and millet) are best for babies of this age. Pour boiling water over them and drain before cooking. 1-year-olds can also be given quinoa, which should be washed and then rinsed in boiling water to remove a somewhat bitter taste. In infrequent cases, there is evidence that glutinous grains (wheat, spelt, and barley, as well as rye, which can be introduced later) can cause coeliac disease. Wait until your baby is at least 6 months old before trying glutinous grains.

All grains should be cooked in water only, without adding salt or sugar. Vary their natural taste by adding fruits or vegetables. A bit of fruit juice mixed with barley cereal is said to improve absorbability of the iron it contains. Wherever possible, we recommend biodynamically grown food. Substitute organic foods if biodynamic products are not available.

When your baby shows increasing interest in the foods you give her to sample, you can begin offering the foods at the beginning of the meal and saving breastfeeding for 'dessert', or vice versa. By the age of 8 months, your baby will become familiar with a whole new palette of foods, and you will know what she likes to eat and can digest without problems.

By this time, your breast milk will begin to decrease and you can start introducing dairy products. Begin by mixing a little mild, natural yoghurt with cereal. When your own milk is reduced to about half of its original amount, about 200 ml (1 US cup) per day of cow's milk is needed to prevent protein or calcium deficiency. As breastfeeding draws to a close, 400 ml (1⅔ US cups) is enough.

A baby who sits in her high chair watching their parents at mealtimes has ample opportunities to gnaw on pieces of apple, carrots and other vegetables, and bread. Your baby's front teeth are adequate for dealing with these foods, but dishes made with unground grains, whether soaked or cooked, should be avoided until molars appear. Meanwhile, cracked grains are better.

Vitamin deficiencies are highly unlikely if your baby's diet includes a variety of fruits, vegetables and grains, even if you use commercial baby foods from time to time. European Union regulations require vitamin enrichment of all cereal foods produced specifically for children between the ages of 5 months and 3 years. For example, all grains and flour products aimed at this age group (cream of rice, spelt cereal, teething biscuits etc.) are enriched with vitamin B$_1$. This is done in order to prevent vitamin deficiencies due to very limited diets. But in developed nations, where a wide variety of foods is readily available, this requirement causes problems for producers committed to providing natural foods. If you want to avoid feeding your baby or toddler foods that contain added vitamins, you can make these items yourself from untreated ingredients or choose brands not intended specifically for small children.

Children are at higher risk of developing allergies if there is a family history of hay fever or food allergies. Breastfeeding exclusively for the first 6 months of your baby's life will reduce the risk. When introducing solid foods to your baby from 6 months onwards, give dairy, eggs, wheat, nuts, seeds, and fish and shellfish one at a time to see if a reaction occurs (if one does, it will be easier to identify the culprit). Do not give your child peanuts before they are 6 months old – and whole nuts until around 5 years old, due to the choking risk.

A longer period of breastfeeding, as currently recommended, is good for the development of your baby's jaw and prevents lazy eating habits, since nursing from the breast takes much more effort than drinking from a bottle. Most fully breastfed babies never use a bottle but simply learn to drink from a cup.

12.15 Infant to toddler

The transition from infant to toddler begins when your baby learns to walk and is able to approach objects on their own. Abandoning crawling in favour of uprightness means that their hands are now free to grasp, tug and examine anything within reach. Being independently mobile puts a totally different face on your baby's daily routine. They can wander off on their own, follow you from room to room, and take their place at the family dinner table. This new situation presents challenges for other members of the family, who must allow the youngest member to participate in age-appropriate ways without making them the constant centre of attention. How and whether this is accomplished establishes a pattern for family interactions at a later age. Children benefit greatly when they experience that their real needs are recognised and respected, their moods are handled with humour and patience, and limits are calmly set when their behaviour is chaotic and demanding.

Your child's sleeping habits also change at this age. In their first year of life, babies nap both in the morning and in the afternoon and have no trouble sleeping outside or near an open window. After age 1, children generally nap only in the afternoon and find it difficult to sleep outdoors or near the window. Give some thought to the timing of your toddler's afternoon nap so she can be outside either before or afterwards and don't spend the nicest part of the day sleeping. Obviously, it will be easier for your child to fall asleep at night if the afternoon nap is earlier rather than later. The more predictable you can make their times for eating and sleeping, the less likely they are to be moody, cranky or at a loose end. Young children like nothing better than fixed habits. Experiencing a regular routine gives children a feeling of security and trust that is reflected in their sense of self (see also Section 13.1) and is the best possible foundation for developing their motivation and will (see page 237).

12.16 Clothing and first shoes

Shoes

Toddlers are very attracted to shoes and love putting them on and taking them off. Later, they identify shoes with the people who wear them and enjoy trying on other people's shoes (and roles).

Initially, however, putting on shoes is difficult. Toddlers tend to curl their toes instead of sticking them straight into the shoe, so it helps to loosen 'beginner' shoes as much as possible before putting them on your child's feet.

Firm-soled shoes are *not* an aid to learning to walk as they make feet passive. For this purpose, going barefoot or wearing socks or soft-soled slippers is better. Outside, grass provides a good surface for your child's first steps; indoors, a natural-fibre carpet provides tactile sensations.

Flat feet are normal in childhood, since foot arches develop only as a result of coming to grips with gravity and usually only after age 4. Children who do not learn to walk do not develop arches. Orthopaedists now agree that truly flat feet, which develop only later, require orthopaedic shoe inserts only in extreme cases that threaten to affect overall posture. In other cases, stimulating independent activity and walking on tiptoes work best. Making a game out of this activity and setting it to a little song or poem works better than conscious demands. Your child is less likely to lose interest if you simply 'fly like a bird' or 'dance on tiptoe like an elf'; as you go through the house, they will imitate and follow you on tiptoe.

The best material for children's shoes is unlined leather. Flat heels are best. Because synthetic or sheepskin fleece linings usually cover only the uppers, not the soles, they are not nearly as effective at keeping feet warm as wool socks, which surround the feet on all sides. Synthetics do not absorb moisture and increase the likelihood of perspiration and athlete's foot. Of course you need to buy shoes large enough to accommodate thick wool socks in winter. Sales staff in shoe stores can help you determine your child's size.

The purpose of shoes is to increase our mobility on rough ground and in bad weather. In puddles or snow and on muddy or gravelly ground, heavy soles with a good tread are best. Soft soles are comfortable on pavements. Children's shoes are available in many styles to meet these different needs.

In summary, the function of shoes is to protect feet from adverse environmental conditions. The healthy shape and function of feet develop through use and activity, not through wearing shoes.

Clothing

Take advantage of your experience during the first few months and years of your child's life. If you have already recognised the advantages of wool, you will continue to avoid synthetics and won't begrudge your preschooler their woolly undershirt. For nightwear for ages 1–4 (or sometimes even 6), a knitted sleeping bag of natural unbleached wool will keep your child evenly warm yet allow them to change position freely. At this age, children are still likely to kick their covers off at night and may not yet be able to cover themselves up again. Your choice of daywear for your child should be based on practicality: that is, freedom of movement, durability, warmth and absorbability. Beyond that, your child's affinity for a special item of clothing can help create the right Sunday or holiday mood.

And what about the colour of clothing? According to Rudolf Steiner, the after-images of colours are what affect us psychologically. When we look at a red surface, a green after-image develops inside us. For an overactive child who tends to 'bang their head against the wall', clothing on the red end of the spectrum can have a harmonising effect by constantly creating an after-image of soothing green. Conversely, dressing a more lethargic or reclusive child predominantly in shades of blue, which create after-images of active yellow and orange, can help stimulate to greater activity. Due to the especially close connection between physical and emotional life in early childhood, your toddler experiences after-images of colour much more intensely than an adult does, and they affect a child's bodily constitution as strongly as any other influences at this age.

12.17 Age-appropriate play and toys

The variety of toys available today is a problem in itself. Children are overwhelmed with commercial products that represent the toy industry's definition of 'age-appropriate', but anyone who has ever observed young children absorbed in play knows how little their activity has to do with what such toys have to offer. Play is a child's natural tendency to become active in their environment. They do whatever they see others do. A 2-year-old will enthusiastically 'stir soup' with a stick on the floor. They want to turn the knobs on the stove like their mother, go 'click' when their father takes a photo, and investigate the plates that come clattering out of the cabinet before supper. What satisfies children most is *activity*, not looking at a perfect plastic doll or a caricature of an animal. But if a doll has no face, or only three dots that suggest a face, their imagination creates the rest. They can make the doll laugh or cry or be angry or tired. Eternally smiling doll faces, or worse still, dolls that 'talk', create false after-images that fixate a child's imagination. Looking into the glass eyes of a teddy bear deadens their own vision.

What makes a toy age-appropriate? In your baby's first year of life, for example, an appropriate toy is a simply made doll consisting of a small piece of silk with the centre filled with wool and tied off to form the head, while the knotted corners become hands. Later, your child can have a wooden doll to stand up and lie down, later still a soft homemade flannel doll. Any object that encourages imaginative activity and is unspecific enough to be used in many different ways is a suitable toy. A toy can be a finger: see how it moves, see everything it can do. It can be the corner of a pillow, to bend and poke inside out. It can be a jar to open and close, to put things into and take them out again. It can be a piece of wood to bang on the table and discover what kind of noise it makes. Later, it may be a water tap, or a bottle cap to scoop up water and fill a pond. A pot and a spoon for drumming are also interesting. So is a colourful knitted ball stuffed with wool, for rolling, throwing and pushing, or small pieces of colourful cloth for covering and uncovering all sorts of things.

It is very important for fathers, mothers, uncles and aunts to give children good toys. Our perfect, rationally conceived modern toys leave no room for a child's imagination, and their materials, colours and shapes usually offend both our sense of reality and our sense of aesthetics. The fascinating, sophisticated movements and optical effects of technological toys turn children into observers instead of active participants. This is particularly true of electronic devices which keep children busy but not in a creative way. However, the most serious issue of playing with such devices is the disturbing effect on healthy brain development. The purpose of play is to provide opportunities for healthy physical development through children's own independent activity and stimulating creative imagination. In his essay *The Education of the Child*, Rudolf Steiner says:

Children learn not by being taught but by imitating. Their physical organs take shape under the influence of their physical surroundings. Healthy vision develops when we ensure that the right colours and lighting are present in the child's surroundings. Similarly, the physical basis of a healthy moral sense develops in the brain and circulatory system when children see morality at work around them. If a child experiences only the foolish actions of others in the first 7 years of her life, her brain will assume forms that make it suited only for foolishness later in life. If we were able to see into the human brain as it develops, we would surely provide our children only with toys that stimulate the brain's formative activity.

Purposeful activity and dexterity are connected with brain development. Speech and language problems are best prevented by play requiring dexterity, balance and spatial awareness.

Developmental perspectives of this sort often conflict with economic interests intent on developing new markets among juvenile consumers. But if families understand what harms and what strengthens children, far-reaching negative impacts such as inner emptiness, apathy and lack of imagination and creativity can be avoided. Many parents today are already beginning to suspect that one important factor in the pervasiveness of drug dependency is the fact that we are taught from a very early age to rely for 'entertainment' on devices that leave no room in our lives for satisfying independent activity and involvement with our surroundings.

12.18 Sleep concerns

Not sleeping through the night

We mentioned earlier that babies sometimes smile briefly in their sleep as if sensing a parent's presence. Similarly, some infants and toddlers open their eyes whenever their father or mother tiptoes into the room, no matter how quietly, but sleep soundly when a sibling is crying loudly right next to them. Sometimes a screaming toddler will calm down if you simply allow them some space and are not anxious about the situation. Conversely, your infant's restlessness increases if you yourself don't know what to do and your thoughts are going around in circles.

The causes of children's sleeping problems are as varied as their manifestations. Below is a list of possibilities to check in each individual case.

Possible causes

- How was your child feeling that day and that evening? Were they outside a lot and did they have enough exercise? Did you notice any physical or emotional symptoms, such as stomach wind, constipation, sweating, chills, jealousy or discontentedness?
- How were you feeling? Were you overtired, unhappy, discontented or working outside the home? Did you feel unappreciated, overstressed or unable to enjoy life? Did you have problems with your in-laws, housemates or neighbours? Were you anxious or worried about the future?
- What about the child's surroundings: the bed, the household, noise, WiFi, radio and television, toys?
- Has your child ever woken during the night for a legitimate but temporary reason that may have become habit? For example, did

you let them sleep in your bed when they were ill?

Some other possibilities are:

• An evening meal that included high-fibre, wind-producing foods.

• Becoming overheated during warm weather.

• A younger sibling who just learned to walk (feelings of jealousy typically appear at this time).

• Constant scolding and prohibitions during the day. For example, do you often have to tell your child to be quiet during the day because you are too concerned about what your neighbours might think?

After considering these different perspectives and coming to a conclusion about why your child can't sleep through the night, the next question is what to do about it. Here are a few recommendations:

The most important but least expected rule for parents is: *Parent's sleep is sacred*. As a parent, you must make sure that you get enough sleep. Without it, you can't possibly put in 16–18-hour days and remain patient and interested. Babies are the last ones to worry about, since it is usually easy for them to make up for lack of sleep.

Do not get up at night more often than absolutely necessary.

You may be able to place the baby's crib next to your bed and reach a hand between the bars when they get restless. Most children fall asleep again as soon as they know that a parent is right there. If there's no room for the crib beside your bed and you can't rearrange your bedroom furniture to accommodate it, sleep on a comfortable mattress in the baby's room.

Toddlers should sleep in a crib; an open bed is impractical because it is much easier for them to bother you if they can get out easily. Reaching one hand into their bed works well until your baby is about 1 year old. After that, a better strategy is to let them see you lying there quietly in the dim light from the street. Outwardly, you are totally quiet and relaxed (try to relax inwardly, too, as best you can manage). Say only once, 'Sleep well, I'm sleeping too.' After that, don't respond to anything your child says or does. After 5 minutes, they'll settle down and go to sleep. Since toddlers are natural imitators, there's nothing else they can do. The situation is totally different if you jump up every time they make a peep. Of course you'll find your child standing straight up in bed and making all the usual demands.

Take your child into your own

bed only as a last resort and only if you yourself are able to sleep under those circumstances. You may want to make an exception to this rule when your child is ill, if they will not overheat. It may be best for the other parent to sleep somewhere else.

Regardless of what you do when your child wakes up at night, only one parent should respond. The disruption is simply multiplied if two adults have their sleep interrupted and have different ideas about what to do next.

At roughly 18 months, when they are learning to talk, children develop an intuitive understanding of the measures their parents are implementing. At this age, they quickly learn to recognise limits, which they could not do before. For example, during a serious illness at age 15 months, one little boy developed the habit of waking up once or twice each night and crying until his mother came to him. By the time the legitimate reasons (discomfort due to illness or thirst due to fever) disappeared, waking up and crying had become a habit.

It is quite normal for children to wake up either fully or partially at some point during the night. This has nothing to do with a real sleep disorder. Some children simply put their thumbs in their mouths and go back to sleep, others just turn over, still others sing themselves to sleep. Some, however, develop the habit of having a parent pick them up, give them bottles and kisses, sing songs and play other little games. By the time this scenario has been repeated every night for 3–5 months, the parent is at the end of their tether and takes the problem to a doctor, who advises them to accommodate the child only to the extent of leaving a door open or night light on, or letting them fall asleep in their own bed before taking them to their own. You can also sleep on a mattress next to your child's bed, or they can sleep in a crib next to yours, but if they wake you up, just state lovingly and firmly: 'Sleep well, I want to sleep, too.'

Even if your child doesn't understand the content of your words, they will sense the mood that lies behind them. That's why it is essential for you to mean what you say. If you're lucky, it will work. If not, you must push your child's crib back into their room and ignore their deafening screams. We know from daily experience that many parents' entire philosophy of bringing up children falls apart at this point. After all, they want the best for their children; they want everything to be beautiful and loving. In reality, however, children become increasingly unhappy, disagreeable and unsatisfied if they never encounter firm limits or sincere intentions. When parents change their tactics and insert rational actions into the parent–child relationship, the child's need for clear limits are satisfied. This is usually impossible without a temporary therapeutic crisis. It is worth it to persist, however, because the consequences of success soon become clearly visible in the child.

The most important rule for implementing any of these measures is to speak with actions, not words. Don't ask, explain or threaten. Often this approach is so foreign to the adults embroiled in such a situation that a conversation with a doctor or health visitor is needed before they can grasp the purpose and importance of such measures. A talk with your doctor is also in order if your partner does not agree on how to proceed or if one of you can't face the turmoil.

Meanwhile, let's imagine the following scenario: You hear your child screaming. You *must* ignore it for 5 minutes, but not for more than 10. When this painful waiting period is over, regardless of whether your child is quiet or still screaming, open the door gently and ask in a friendly tone of voice, 'Are you ready to be quiet?'

and if they are outside their bedroom, take them back inside (or to wherever you want them to sleep). But if your child's screaming intensifies, say, 'When you're ready, I'll come back' and then shut the door. Repeat the procedure after another 5 minutes: again, regardless of whether your child is quiet or screaming. Your conciliatory attitude is important. If you have been inconsistent in the past, not doing what you said you would do, the torment will continue for a while, but after a couple of repetitions an 18-month-old usually understands that there's nothing to be gained from more crying. You may need to stand beside their bed and put up with their screaming for a bit. The important thing is that your reaction is now calm and deliberate – totally different from how you used to behave. No 'calming' flood of words, no despairing 'Oh, poor baby', no picking them up, no kiss; maybe just a little quiet humming or singing. If all of this doesn't work in 5 minutes, go out and shut the door and start over again. The atmosphere will be intense, because you want your child to get to the point where you can say, 'Good, now you're ready.'

From the very beginning, your attitude must be conciliatory, but you must not abandon the objective, necessary limit you've decided on. The next night, calling out to your child to be quiet (again, in a friendly tone of voice) is usually enough. You should be quite sure, however, that your child isn't coming down with an infection – a legitimate reason for crying – just as you begin to insist on a change of habits. And it makes no sense to shut the door if they can open it; you might consider placing a temporary barrier such as a stair gate over the door.

The bad habit of giving your child a bottle in bed makes the situation more difficult. It helps to simply place the usual bottle or cup of water (or herb tea) nearby, without giving it to them. Your child may sleep through without needing to drink if their 'slave' doesn't hand them the bottle. Or tell your child cheerfully one day, 'You're so big now, you don't need a bottle any more. Instead, this little gnome will tell you a story if you wake up,' or something similar. Knitted woollen gnomes are especially suitable sleeping companions at this age (See *The Gnome Craft Book*, page 332). They can also comfort sick children and are sometimes even an acceptable substitute for having a parent around all the time.

Bedtime fusses and trouble falling asleep

Like children who wake up at night, little ones who have trouble falling asleep often fuss simply out of habit. Changing your child's bedtime ritual can be the basis for drawing new, helpful limits. For example:

- Hang a blue cloth with a couple of gold stars on the wall or over your child's bed to make a 'starry sky'.
- A new sleeping companion – maybe the above-mentioned gnome – may appear to wish your child good night.
- By candlelight, sing a song or play a piece on a children's harp or recorder.

If you've been doing all this, it might be time to abandon these habits and try something new and fun that may even take a bit more time. Being allowed to stay up a little longer and hear a brief story as they sit on the sofa with you will make your child feel grown-up and privileged. After the story, though, it is definitely time for bed.

When your child gets up and comes out of their room for the first time, calmly take her back to bed and tell her that you're going to shut the door if she comes out again. The second time, shut the door – equally calmly, of course.

If your child can turn the light on by herself, disconnect the fuse as a pre-emptive measure, but make sure the blinds let in a bit of light from outside. Use the 5-minute wait as described above. The door stays open only when your child stays in bed.

Children are smart – by the second evening, they will accept the new limits. These measures actually fail only when parents don't have the courage to carry out the consequences they've decided upon – which is deeply disappointing to the children.

A different type of difficulty in falling asleep is due to nervousness; your child somehow gets the idea that they can't fall asleep. There are any number of different possible causes: being overtired, hot weather, excitement, knowing that you're going away, the start of a vacation. In this case, try singing a song or giving your child something of yours – perhaps a sweater or the blanket from your bed – to keep in bed with them. Tuck them in again and stroke their hair to comfort them. Sometimes the best tactic may be to let children come into the living room for a bit and look at a book by themselves. Say something like, 'When you're tired, you can just put yourself back to bed.' In this case, of course, you must avoid carrying on a conversation with them and be visibly involved in activities that have nothing to do with them. Boredom, together with pride in being old enough to know when they are tired, will usually send your child back to bed soon.

Sleeping disorders at school age

Before going to sleep, check your child's feet are warm (if necessary give them a hot-water bottle or have them wear socks), or have a warm bath with bath oils like lavender. Sometimes a walk around the block to get some fresh air helps.

See that the evening meal is not too heavy: not too many fats, nor too many uncooked vegetables or grains. Warm milky semolina or similar can help, as can herbal tea with a little honey. Read a story aloud, rather than letting your child read themselves. Take a few minutes to discuss the events of the day or, if your child has worries, the coming day. This is also important if you are worried and your child senses this. It helps to be clear about the forthcoming events. A short comforting word, such as 'We'll manage it together', can give peace of mind.

Nocturnal fears

Sudden screaming at night can have a variety of causes, different in

6–18-month-olds than in 3-year-olds. The first time this symptom appears, check whether your child is wide awake or screaming in their sleep because of a bad dream. If the latter, cuddle them or wake them up gently. Then check for signs of pain (such as a hard abdomen), fever or difficulty breathing through their nose. Finally, try to recall whether your child had a frightening experience that day. Did you notice any unusual fearfulness? Your own assessment of the symptoms will determine whether you need to consult your doctor.

Children with 'night terrors' scream or moan in their sleep or toss and turn in bed and can neither wake up immediately nor go back to sleeping peacefully. Here, too, be alert for unusual events during the day and foods that might cause wind. Restlessness that reappears at 4-week intervals may be related to lunar phases. In most cases, anthroposophic or homeopathic medications are very effective, for instance Arsenicum album 12X, 5–10 globules, 1–3 times a day.

Sleepwalking

Sleepwalking, which occurs most frequently at full moon, can be dangerous if the sleepwalker wakes up while wandering around. This symptom also responds to the types of anthro-posophic or homeopathic medications mentioned above. As with nocturnal anxiety, psychotropic drugs are not necessary.

12.19 Toilet training

In the second year of life, children's digestive systems are challenged to the utmost because they still chew poorly but want to try everything edible. The intervals between bowel movements may vary tremendously and their stools, which may make a mess up to their shoulder blades several times a day, look undigested and usually smell sour. If your child seems otherwise well and does not lose weight, there is no need for concern. Regular meal-times and restricting bloating or laxative foods such as coarse oat flakes, whole or coarsely ground grains, and raw foods will help your child's digestion somewhat. Urination becomes less frequent; the quantity of urine increases and it develops a stronger odour.

For convenience, most parents switch to disposable nappies when their babies become independently mobile, but some experienced parents (imagining the resulting mountain of rubbish) continue to have success with cloth nappies, wool soakers and babygrows. This combination keeps the stools adequately contained, the smell signals when a nappy change is due, and the baby's skin stays fresh. Because toddlers urinate less frequently but in larger quantities, they soon begin to indicate when they need changing, so they are less likely to stay wet for long periods and problems of evaporative cooling and skin irritation recede into the background. At this stage, too, you are more likely to recognise the critical times in advance and change your child's nappies promptly.

Systematic attempts at toilet training should not play a role until the third or even fourth year. The simplest process is to remove your child's nappy between meals and place a potty on the floor for your child to use. The more unselfconsciously and routinely this process is managed, the better, regardless of when your child ultimately becomes toilet trained. The less emphasis you place on toilet training as such, the more likely it is that your child will learn to use the toilet as a matter of course.

12.20 Bedwetting

If bedwetting continues until age 4, your child should be examined by a paediatrician. The causes may be either constitutional, physical or psychological. The measures discussed below are helpful when physical causes have been ruled out.

The first step is to look for shocks, reasons for jealousy, after-effects of illness and the like. Once these issues are clarified, it is usually worth trying to accommodate your child's need for more protection and comfort. Allow them to be 'little' and 'protected' again for a while by consciously reverting to old habits from earlier childhood. Meanwhile, try to make the course of the day more regular and consistent and carry your child in your consciousness more than you would otherwise. At the preschool age, do not address the bedwetting situation directly; instead, look for other ways to solve the problem.

When a younger sibling is born or has just learned to walk – events that could make you pay less attention to your older child – give them an extra big hug to help them share your joy in this event. Show your older child that you are proud of them for being so big. To differentiate their drinking vessel from the baby's, give them a special new drinking cup or special silverware of their own – without commenting on it.

If your child is used to hearing stories you make up, they can include symbolic representations of bedwetting, such as a flooded brook or overflowing spring that people have to control with a child's help. Or tell them about an old man who has to struggle every day with the sluice that controls the water level in a fishpond until a child comes along and helps him or takes over the job.

Punishing bedwetting simply intensifies your child's need for more attention and makes the condition worse. If your child feels accommodated and appreciated, however, some extra attentiveness on your part will eliminate the problem. For example, if children regularly wet the bed at 10:30 pm and 6:00 am, accompany them on their last trip to the bathroom before bedtime and encourage them to do a 'nice big pee'. An hour or two after they go to bed, watch for signs of restlessness; if you suspect their bladder is full, take them to the bathroom, put them on the toilet and say a few quiet, encouraging words. Do the same thing at 6:00 am (if it doesn't mean you lose too much sleep; you'll need to wake up before your child does). These efforts on your part mean that you accept part of the responsibility for keeping your child dry. Watch for the right time to give this responsibility back to your child. This method doesn't work for children who wet the bed at unpredictable times during the night or who resist your efforts to wake them. It is also of questionable value if your child sleeps so soundly they don't notice they're wet. In that case, you'll need to decide whether to resort to nappies at night or whether a rubber mattress protector is enough.

A consistent daily routine, especially with regard to eating and drinking habits, will help strengthen your child's constitution. If you're not willing to establish a regular rhythm for what goes in, you can't expect regularity in what comes out. Attempting to treat bedwetting makes no sense if your child is a non-stop or 'on demand' drinker. In this case, the first step is to restrict drinking to meal and snack times, when you can control the quantities.

It is important to dress children who wet the bed warmly in wool underwear or tights (heavier or lighter, depending on the season) that cover as much of their torso as possible. If their feet get wet and cold, give them a warm footbath and rub their feet with massage oil, red copper ointment or solum oil afterwards. Rubbing their legs with St John's wort oil in the mornings also helps.

Finally, make sure that children see enough activities that are worth imitating and challenge them to develop further. The feeling of 'coasting along in neutral' encourages children to regress to earlier stages of development. Other triggers, such as conflict at home, absent parents or an impending divorce usually indicate that a talk with a child psychologist or paediatrician is needed.

Assuming that physical causes have been ruled out, the same measures apply if your child wets during the day as well as at night. You will also need to set an 'internal alarm clock' for your child during the day, which is exactly what you do with a younger child who is learning to stay dry. Introduce new toilet habits, such as specific times for sitting on the toilet or the potty, without talking about the situation.

The cause of 'leakage' and damp underwear also needs to be clarified. Often this is simply a sign of inattentiveness. If that's the case, accompany children to the toilet whenever possible and encourage them to fully empty their bladder – but abandon this tactic if your child enjoys this type of attention too much.

Once children are 7 or 8 years old, a different approach is appropriate. Once they are ready for school, they are also ready and willing to listen to adults they respect and trust, such as teachers, godparents, doctors and so on. Direct reproaches, however, are still too much for them. A time-tested method is for an adult confidant to tell a little story that mentions wetting directly. For example:

At night, there's a little gnome (or a bird or a fairy, as you like) on your shoulder who stays awake while you sleep and whispers secretly in our ear, 'Wake up, you need to go to the bathroom.' But you just lie there and don't hear anything, even though he's trying so hard to help you. Try paying really close attention at night and see if you can hear him. If you do, you'll wake up and go quietly to the bathroom. You just have to decide to do that before you go to sleep. Your mother will remind you about it when she says good night.

The person telling the story then asks you to whisper mysteriously in your child's ear each evening, 'Don't forget to listen to the little gnome!' It is usually less effective if a parent tells this story.

This approach works because

your child really doesn't want to wet the bed any more. The gnome, bird or fairy becomes a symbol of their intention to wake up, which is still not strong enough. Allowing this symbolic image to grow in your child's consciousness by reminding them every evening can help strengthen their weak intentions and make it easier for them to wake up.

Children of this age are still too young for direct admonishments. 'Appealing to their conscience' is appropriate only after age 9, when it is also more effective for a third party (the child's doctor is the best choice) to implement the treatment. Sometimes a temporary change of scenery is helpful because it strengthens children's self-awareness and forces them to rely on themselves more. Depending on your child's constitution and maturity, it may also be possible to train their bladder by deliberately increasing the time between trips to the bathroom. At this stage, it is good for children to determine their own schedule of eating and drinking.

Using a bedwetting alarm may also work, but usually only in combination with a parent who will cheerfully supervise the trip to the bathroom.

12.21 Soiling

By soiling, we mean that your child deliberately poos their pants or in a corner of the room. This is different from the dirty pants of a constipated or forgetful child, which simply need humorous attention on your part and increased efforts to adapt your daily routine to your child's bowel habits. Very few readers of this book will ever encounter true soiling (encopresis). Occasional soiling is usually a consequence of turbulent interpersonal situations and a sign that the child is either looking for a way out, testing their parents, or afraid of an unfamiliar toilet or potty seat. These situations are easy to recognise and correct. Soiling that persists for weeks and months, however, is always a sign of resignation on the part of both the child and her parents, and in most cases stopping it is unlikely without outside help. Anyone with connections to the family should encourage the parents to contact a paediatrician, child psychiatrist or family counselling centre.

12.22 Thumb sucking

When children suck their thumb, they are sealed off from the outer world and feel comfortably self-contained. If you pull a 2-year-old thumb-sucker's thumb out of their mouth, it pops right back in as if attached to an invisible spring. If you hold it to prevent it from going back in, the child will awaken reluctantly from their dreamy state and acknowledge the intrusion with displeasure. But if they hear you scraping pudding off the bottom of a saucepan or getting the stroller ready for a walk, their thumb will pop out by itself at these tempting sounds, and if you tried to get them to put it back in their mouth, they would resist as vehemently as they do when you try to make them stop sucking it.

Specially shaped dummies are often recommended by some doctors because deep penetration during thumb sucking is known to cause jaw deformation. However, jaw deformation due to thumb sucking often reverses itself spontaneously when the permanent teeth begin to emerge and thumb sucking gradually stops. In any case, a thumb (or other fingers) in the mouth is not the only cause of jaw deformation. We have also seen cases due to dummy use.

We advise against dummies because they encourage children to suck even when they would not do so spontaneously. And because a dummy on a string around your child's neck is always available, it can easily be misused to keep them quiet or independently occupied or to deceive them into thinking that food is on the way. A thumb, although also always available, is preferable because it has a self-renewing surface that is less susceptible to fungal contamination, and children will never keep their thumb in their mouth when they want to play actively. If you do decide to give your child a dummy, do not fasten it around their neck; use a dummy clip to attach it to their clothing (ensure the cord is short enough that it cannot become looped around their neck).

Some of our readers will surely ask whether this means it is best to do nothing at all about thumb sucking. We recommend not trying to stop children from sucking their thumb before they fall asleep at night. For daytime thumb sucking, patience is often the best approach. 5-year-olds sometimes decide from one day to the next that they are done with thumb sucking forever and actually stick to their decision. One mother even noticed her child's hand jerking away from his mouth as he slept. On the other hand, if your 3-year-old develops a callus on their thumb, a bandage may help break the habit earlier. Cover the callus with ointment and gauze, secure the thumb bandage with a gauze strip tied around your child's wrist, and cover the entire hand with a little cloth sack. Your child will be astonished at the changed appearance of this extremity; be calm and tell them that everything is just fine. Change the bandage daily for a week and then leave it off. By then, your child may have forgotten about sucking their thumb. *Do not* use adhesive bandages, which can be swallowed.

Thumb sucking indicates the persistence of an earlier developmental stage (nursing), so neither forbidding nor encouraging thumb sucking are appropriate responses. If you sense your child needs more of the physical self-perception that nursing once supplied, you can help them by lovingly stroking their head as they fall asleep or by encouraging active interaction with their surroundings.

13. Promoting Health and Preventing Illness

For the last 300 years, the question of how disease develops dominated medical discussion, and prevention was understood as avoiding harmful influences and risk factors. For instance, during a flu epidemic that sickens 15% of the population, why are the remaining 85% not infected? What bodily, psychological or spiritual factors are ultimately responsible for the immunological strength that results in their remaining unaffected?

In the second half of the twentieth century a new, health-oriented approach to medical research was developed, called salutogenesis (from the Latin *salus*, 'health', and *genesis*, 'creation': understanding how to maintain health and prevent illness in connection with medicine and education.

By preventative paediatric medicine, we mean first of all regular medical check-ups, officially recommended immunisations, prevention of tooth decay and rickets, and the basics of nutrition and general hygiene. But we also hear questions such as, how does ultrasound affect the growing embryo?

This question is a good example of how disease prevention and health promotion interact. During an ultrasound exam (sonography), sound waves with frequencies above the range of human hearing are sent out as either pulses or continuous sound. Tissues treated with ultrasound produce characteristic echo waves that are then captured and made visible through computer technology. When these mechanically produced sound waves meet living tissues, we cannot say for certain that they have no effect, even if no damage has ever been proven in the 40 years since the introduction of this technology. The only good rule is *as little as possible, as much as necessary.* If this rule was followed it would be an important step towards a more health-oriented approach. What causes harm and what promotes health is always a question of both degree and reciprocal compensation.

13.1 A holistic approach to working with illness

Rudolf Steiner described human beings as functioning across four levels:

- *The physical body*, which facilitates movement and sensory perception.
- *The life (or etheric) body*, which facilitates life processes of growth and self-healing.
- *The soul (or astral) body*, which facilitates the experience of emotions and behaviour.
- *The spirit (self or 'I') body*, which facilitates the experiences of consciousness, personality, identity and will.

Children come to the world as soul-spiritual beings with the task of 'incarnating' into their bodies and learning to feel at home there. The more suitable the body (or the more suitable it becomes as the child develops), the easier this process is. How many people today feel like strangers to themselves because they are not totally comfortable in their bodies or cannot express themselves through them? The role of medicine and education is to create conditions that permit the healthiest possible incarnation process.

Childhood illnesses play an important part in working through and individualising specific parts of the body. The thrust of the symptoms of childhood diseases may be directed either outwards (as in skin symptoms) or inwards (in the diseases involving the blood or individual organs). The body's response to each illness is a one-sided or unbalanced activity summoned up by the child's 'I' in an effort to alter the interaction across the different levels of their constitution.

Illnesses with *high fevers*, like scarlet fever, measles or roseola, are primarily an indication that the 'I' and its warmth activity are intervening in functions of the life body, influencing metabolic processes more strongly than usual and triggering fever-induced immune processes.

Children with *whooping cough*, on the other hand, takes possession of their body's respiratory organs and functions in a new way, allowing the soul body to work strongly.

Diseases that involve significant *swelling of lymph nodes or glands* allow children to get a new grip on their life body processes, making it more active.

The water-filled blisters of *chickenpox* contain endogenous matter that needs to be eliminated. These blisters and the subsequent development of small scars subtly alter the child's physical form.

If we attribute symptoms exclusively to germs and recovery to the disappearance of pathogens, the most important questions remain unanswered.

- What is the relationship between a particular illness and the being of this patient?
- Why does the illness affect someone else differently or not at all?
- What is the relationship between the pathogen and the essential nature of the illness?

The medical histories of different individuals are never exactly the same. One had a bad case of measles but a mild case of scarlet fever, the other the opposite. One person never contracted whooping cough, another never had mumps. Individual differences of this sort reveal something about the nature of the person in question, something we ordinarily fail to consider. But how do we develop susceptibility to a particular illness?

13.2 How does health develop?

Medical sociologist Aaron Antonovsky lists three main causes of the development and persistence of health.[6] Their three primary factors involve the ability to be resilient, whether on the level of the body, the soul or the spirit:

1. *Overcoming heterostasis, that is, metabolic imbalances resulting from nutrition, movement, rest, climate change and other disturbances.* Each body, organ and individual cell is located somewhere on a continuum of health and illness. New health develops constantly as disruptive factors and pathological tendencies are overcome.

2. *Building up what is called the 'sense of coherence' during childhood and adolescence.* What Antonovsky means is the possibility of processing everything we encounter in a meaningful way and integrating it into a personal sense of our own life and understanding of our environment. The more meaningfully the different levels of experience (as well as each new experience) can be incorporated into an evolving overall picture, the healthier the person and the more resilient and inspiring their. outlook on life.

3. *Using 'resistance resources' (resilience) to come to grips with the stresses and adversities of life.* Resilience represents an individual's sum total of compensation and coping strategies for

positively overcoming problems and worries in life and work. These resources help prevent people from completely breaking down under overwork, anxiety, stress or that they only recover with great difficulty from such a breakdown.

Those in special education refer to 'resilience research', the study of factors that make children resistant and able to grow up healthy in spite of domestic situations marked by chaos, alcoholism, violence or other stress factors. Decisive factors that preserve and enhance resistance include:

- Being loved by another person.
- Believing in God.
- Trusting in progress and in the future.
- Being able to find meaning in one's own destiny by processing problems and conflicts and integrating them into one's life.
- Outer security and a high standard of living.
- A stable social network.

If health is the body's ability to balance out one-sided stress factors and counteract possible disease tendencies, there must be as many different forms of 'health' as there are of illness. Individuals face unique and specific challenges in regulating body heat, ensuring adequate supplies of oxygen and nutrients, and establishing a fragile state of balance between breakdown and regeneration processes in the body. These efforts require just as much care and support as children's emotional and mental ability to process events.

13.3 Hygiene and the immune system

In the bacteriological sense, hygiene includes thoroughly washing hands and kitchen utensils and ensuring the safety of water and food. Without consistent implementation of such hygienic measures, the successes of epidemic control would have been impossible, and rates of infant and maternal mortality would still be at nineteenth-century levels.

Nonetheless, every mother knows that their well-protected baby on the changing table will soon be crawling around on floors dirtied by other people's shoes. In the long run, the immune system is strengthened by use, not by avoidance. Our bodies must learn to cope with germs, and at the same time let them build up their own healthy environment, the microbiome. Country children are often healthier than city children because they are exposed to a multiplicity of influences from nature and the environment both earlier and longer.

It is also important to consider whether every bacterial illness should be treated with antibiotics or only those that a child is unable to overcome without such help. Experience shows that first children are seldom ill as babies because they grow up alone and catch infections only from their parents. When they enter kindergarten, however, we can expect at least two winters of frequent colds. First children bring home almost every infection that is going around; they seem to spend more time at home than in kindergarten.

Second children have similar experiences, but by the time third children come along, they constantly catch upper respiratory infections from their older siblings and may also come down with alarmingly severe cases of the classic childhood diseases at very early ages. These third children, however, are often the sturdiest and healthiest later on.

13.4 Counselling and meditation

The following are examples of what adults can do both for themselves and indirectly, by modelling health-promoting behaviours, for their children.

The most important and readily available means of preventing illness is to **enjoy your work**. It generates emotional warmth that keeps the body healthy. Thus it is essential to organise or approach your daily work in ways that make it possible for you to enjoy it.

Anger, quarrelling, agitation, chronic stress and the lack of a sense of coherence and connection are not only psychologically unsettling but also undermine health. Almost everyone is aware of this type of **psychosocial stress** from direct personal experience. Over longer periods of time, taking unprocessed influences of this sort into sleep means that sleep loses its revitalising effect. We feel less refreshed in the morning and become more susceptible to infectious diseases.

This combination of personal and social problems can be effectively dealt with by deciding to pursue either a path of self-development or conflict resolution methods. **Psychotherapy, biography work and pastoral counselling** offer many different options. **Anthroposophic meditative training** also offers techniques for meditation, concentration and relaxation.

Although their *raison dětre* is

the search for self-knowledge and a spiritual understanding of the world rather than the preservation of health, these techniques, like all other sincere spiritual efforts, have direct positive effects on health. For example, the beneficial ordering effects of Steiner's verbal meditations are immediately apparent on reading them. It is helpful to recall and reflect on words and themes of this sort now and again in the course of the day or before important or difficult events.

We are fully justified in thinking of hygiene not only as regular bathing, clean clothes and appropriate living conditions but also in terms of emotional and mental hygiene. Do we cultivate our life of soul and spirit as carefully as we care for our bodies? Couldn't a brief session of meditation or concentration exercises each morning and evening become just as much of a need as brushing our teeth? Rudolf Steiner's discussions of nervousness and the human 'I' and of practical training in thought offer a series of very effective exercises for schooling attentiveness, memory, perception and concentration.[7]

Other central issues of emotional hygiene include how we think and feel about other people and realising that our thoughts and feelings can be either destructive or constructive for ourselves and for others. How we think and feel contributes to the 'climate' in our homes, which is also experienced and judged by our children and teenagers.

13.5 The powerful effects of art

Artistic activity is a very gratifying way of promoting health. Again, we have Steiner's research to thank for providing an exact scientific basis for this field.

Modelling therapy

The creative activity of modelling, sculpting and carving directly stimulates and regulates the sculptural, formative functioning of the life body (see page 237), to which it corresponds.

Painting therapy

Handling colour tones and moods in painting harmonises the collaboration between the life and soul bodies.

Drawing geometric forms or objects in perspective awakens forces of structure and form. Rhythmical form-drawing directly influences respiration and heartbeat. When layers of dilute water colours are applied to the painting surface with rhythmical brush strokes, shapes and transparent layers of colours slowly begin to appear. If the soul follows this process, it lingers in the flow between movement and form and delights in the bright colours. Head and thoughts become free and unburdened or challenged to concentrate and become structured. Feelings find an outlet or are awakened in the experience of colour. Actions are planned and pondered or implemented spontaneously and afresh.

Success makes the painter feel emotionally balanced and well, right down into the physical element: cold and warmth processes are regulated, along with respiration. The painter's experimental, searching, discovering and researching attitude is always in the foreground, in order to develop new perspectives in the process of creating. The point here is to be active, to take hold and intervene, to transform, to try out, to risk throwing everything away and starting over again. Or to rest, to arrive, to be self-contained and enjoy the colours.

Music therapy

Musical laws and their relationship to air (as the vehicle of sound) corresponds to the activity of the soul body, which is also musical in character. Every detail of the human body is structured according to specific proportions and numbers, not only with regard to the body's shape but also the rhythms and relative proportions of its physiological functions.

In the book *The Harmony of the Human Body*, Armin Husemann makes a first attempt at a comprehensive understanding of the musical laws governing the human body. Singing and other musical activity, but also working with different colour 'tones' and moods in painting, has harmonising effects on soul activity. The result is a sense of emotional harmony that works back on bodily functions.

Speech therapy

Through artistic speech and speech therapy, the 'I' is directly activated. After all, we express ourselves in the truest sense of the word when we say something about ourselves or how we understand the world.

13.6 Curative eurythmy

The art of eurythmy, pioneered by Rudolf Steiner from 1911 to 1924 and developed further after his death, consists of movements and forms that correspond to specific elements of speech and music. Eurythmy, which is based on an exact understanding of the qualities of individual speech sounds and tones, studies vowels and consonants, pitches and intervals, in relationship to the human form. The gestures corresponding to sounds and tones are the same as the movements that can be observed in the embryo, both in the development of body proportions and in the flowing forms of blood and tissue fluids: growth and holding back, extension and involution, expansion and contraction, enclosure and exclusion, touching and penetration.

Eurythmy's basic gestures encompass all of the human organism's potential movements as well as all movements in the living and unenlivened natural world. We find these gestures repeated in the various growth forms of plants and animals and in the play of movements on surfaces where solids, fluids and gases meet. For this reason, eurythmy can be described as a visible archetypal language in which nature and human beings express their messages through gestures. All forms can be interpreted as movements come to rest; eurythmy makes their development visible and thus offers possibilities for self-education, a means of feeling our way into the development of visible natural shapes.

In *artistic eurythmy*, poems, stories, dramatic works and musical compositions for one or more voices (up to and including entire orchestral pieces) are practised and presented on stage either by individuals or by ensembles.

In *educational eurythmy*, students from kindergarten to twelfth grade learn to move skilfully and orient themselves in space. By practising artistic works, they learn to shape their movements in ways that express a great variety of soul experiences. Doing eurythmy in a group also fosters social skills by allowing youngsters to experience that the success of a major artistic presentation depends entirely on selfless individual contributions.

In *curative eurythmy*, repeated practice of specific speech sounds and tone exercises stimulate formative and regenerative activity in the body and counteract pathological changes. The speed or intensity of individual exercises is adapted to enhance or restrain formative impulses in the body as needed. Other specific exercises have harmonising, stimulating, concentration-promoting or calming effects. For isolated learning disabilities, specific exercises in dexterity, spatial awareness and symmetry are helpful. Curative eurythmy is also helpful in treating movement, hearing and visual disorders because it helps the child's soul penetrate the body more completely. Specific exercises are prescribed by a physician in consultation with the child's teacher and the curative eurythmist.

13.7 Cultivating healthy rhythms

In early childhood, it is especially important to cultivate healthy rhythms because the infant's ability to regulate rhythmic functions is still undeveloped and needs support and stimulation.

The circumstances of modern life and work often encourage us to disregard essential rhythms. This disregard promotes a number of different illnesses or weakened states. Eventually, years or decades of flouting natural rhythms may result in exhaustion and collapse. In contrast, consciously cultivating the most important rhythms, like regular sufficient sleep, increases the body's stress tolerance and prepares it to encounter life's challenges.

What is so special about rhythm?

'Rhythm is the carrier of life,' was the answer Rudolf Steiner gave Rudolf Hauschka when asked what life was.

Rhythm is the repetition of similar processes under comparable circumstances. In respiration, the archetypal rhythm, no breath is exactly as deep or as long as any other, if measured exactly, and yet each breath is similar to the last.

Every rhythm balances out polarities. Wherever contrasting elements collide in nature, rhythms mediate between them. For example, rhythmically structured fleecy clouds appear in the sky where high and low pressure systems meet. Rhythmical wave patterns line the shore, where movable water encounters solid ground. The breathing process mentioned above rhythmically balances the polarities of movement and rest.

Rhythms form the basis of every adaptive process. Rhythmical repetitions are never exactly the same but represent subtle fluctuation around an average value, making them adaptable and flexible, whereas a strict tempo is totally inflexible and has no capacity for balancing out or integrating differences.

Rhythm substitutes for strength. Any rhythmically repeated action takes less exertion and energy than a one-time action performed at an unusual time or under unusual circumstances.

Regular, rhythmical activities foster the development of habits, which are the structure underlying personality and character. Learning to observe regular times for eating and sleeping and to structure the day in a way that balances work and recreation, tension and relaxation, allows us to face the demands of daily life reliably and productively. In contrast, when we pay no attention to our internal clocks and become heavily dependent on outer circumstances or on our own momentary inclinations, we risk exhausting ourselves because we overestimate what we can accomplish. We lack the flexibility to adapt, the strength to persevere and a sense of healthy limits.

Rhythms link nature and humans to the change of seasons, the sequence of day and night, and the many different movements of the planets against the background of the fixed stars. All of the rhythms that regulate the courses of the planets in our solar system are reflected in the life processes of plants, animals and humans and reveal the common origin and connected life of all known creation.

Only in the twentieth century did research on biological rhythms and time structures become a recognised branch of science. The sections that follow provide an overview of the essential rhythms that underlie and support life processes.

Our suggestions on daily, weekly, monthly and yearly rhythms are intended to stimulate a new family culture that once again takes these rhythms into account. Healthier, more adaptable children are our reward for our efforts.

In the past few centuries, human beings have become increasingly emancipated from the rhythms of weeks, months and seasons and now often experience how lack of rhythm and time have undermined our health, leading to 'burnout' with its increased irritability and sense of powerlessness. 'Having time' begins with consciously cultivating time, in other words, with rhythmically shaping its sequences and intervals by alternating different activities and building in breaks.

The same is true of cultivating spiritual and meditative activity: inner work regularly distributed over daily or longer rhythms is the secret to planting the seeds of inner forces and capabilities and fostering their development.

Daily rhythms

Newborns have not yet learned to develop a rhythmic alternation between day and night. Their fluctuations in body temperature (0.5°C/1°F lower in the morning than in the evening), blood sugar levels, levels of various hormones and blood salts and other metabolic processes are not yet synchronised with the sun.

The later structure, elasticity and adaptability of a person's rhythmic system depend on how it is imprinted in infancy with all of daily life's little actions related to eating, bathing, playing and sleeping. All organs, especially the large organs of metabolism and digestion, must coordinate their functions and learn how to work together optimally.

Advice on structuring a baby's daily routine

The more clearly a baby's day takes shape in the course of the first weeks and months – for example, mornings at home, afternoons spent outside being carried in a sling – the more strongly he will experience the course of the day and the difference between day and night and be able to respond with their entire body.

- Create regular alternations between activity and sleep, eating and not eating.
- Pay special attention to getting up in the morning and going to bed at night (always at approximately the same time, if possible).
- In the morning, sing a song and look out of the window together.
- From the very beginning, an infant's bedtime ritual can include lighting a candle, singing a few notes, a short evening story or prayer and a good-night kiss.

Weekly rhythm

The names of the days of the week reflect the fact that they were once associated with the planets including the Sun and Moon that moved across the background of fixed stars. The planets in the sky are very different in their individual manifestations. With practice, we can become aware that the days of the week are equally different in character.

Chronobiology and research on rhythms has shown that the 7-day rhythm is the essential rhythm underlying responsive processes, including adaptation and healing. Acknowledging the rhythmic character of the course of the week is a way to support and stabilise the 7-day rhythm as the basis for flexible reactions to stresses and injuries of all kinds.

Advice on cultivating a weekly routine

- Start every day with a special morning song.
- The 'working' days or school days of the week may have specific, repeated activities. Such regular commitments, distributed well throughout the week to avoid becoming overtired, can be anticipated with pleasure and set the tone for each day.
- Plan your meals based on a weekly pattern.
- Weekends can feel more relaxed, with a more leisurely breakfast, and relaxed family activities, such as singing together or reading aloud.

Monthly rhythms

From the science of climatotherapy, we know that the restorative value of a 4-week cure is significantly greater than that of a 2- or 3-week cure. And when someone is truly exhausted, 2–3 months of recuperation are needed; a 4-week vacation is not enough. The monthly rhythm of the Moon is deeply connected to human physiology, even if it is only apparent in menstruation.

The monthly rhythm is also seen in profound recuperation, habit development and stabilisation. It takes at least 4 weeks for a new habit to take hold. Waldorf Schools take advantage of this fact by dividing instruction into 4-week subject blocks whenever possible.

In planning your vacation, we urge you to consider the 4-week rhythm whenever possible. We advise against short vacations when rest and relaxation are the goal. Short breaks may be a stimulating change of pace for adults, but they are more likely to be a strain on children, who often come down with infections during or after a short vacation.

The rhythm of the year

It takes 9 months of gestation plus the first 3 months after birth for infants' physical bodies to mature to the point where they can focus their eyes and grasp with their hands. It takes another year for them to learn to walk, another to learn to speak and still another year until independent thinking begins. The physical body continues to develop in yearly rhythms, and seasonal changes in weather and light stimulate bodily changes. Similarly, each childhood illness has specific years of life in which cases are most and least likely to occur.

Long-term adaptation also follows yearly rhythms. When we have lived for more than one year in the same place, we feel at home there. When we have lived there for more than seven years, we feel like locals.

Advice on cultivating an annual rhythm

- Looking at calendar pictures.
- Singing songs about the months.
- Observing seasonally changing natural processes and related farm and garden work.
- The type of clothing we wear also changes as the months go by.
- It is a good tradition to celebrate the anniversaries of historical events, just as we celebrate birthdays and yearly seasonal festivals and holidays.

13.8 Constitutional treatment

How is an individual constituted in health and in sickness? How does their bodily and emotional constitution reveal itself?

The anthroposophical view of the human being distinguishes four layers of being (or 'members', as Rudolf Steiner called them) of the human constitution (see Section 13.1, page 237): bodily form and movement (physical body); life processes, such as growth (life or etheric body); emotions and behaviour (soul or astral body); and personality or self (spirit or 'I' body). Also at work in the human constitution is the functional division into three systems: the sensory-nervous system, the rhythmical functions of respiration and circulation; and metabolic functions.

If any of these layers of being or functional systems lapse into one-sidedness, it can cause predisposition to illness, which can then be modulated by constitutional treatments (or therapy).

Since this book repeatedly mentions where a constitutional treatment may be warranted and what it may accomplish, we will introduce some of the basic principles here. **Any course of constitutional therapy should always be discussed with and/ or prescribed by a doctor.** Classical homeopathy uses the term 'constitutional therapy' or 'constitutional treatment' when treating a specific unfavourable basic predisposition with the remedy most appropriate to its clinical picture. *Similia similibus curentur* or 'like cures like' is the homeopathic treatment principle at work here. Anthroposophic doctors often also apply this homeopathic approach to constitutional treatment.

In many cases, the only

differences may be that anthroposophic medicine does not use high potencies (none over 30X) and that the duration and dosage of treatment differs because here too the unique rhythms of the constitutional layers of being (members) are also taken into account, as described by Rudolf Steiner in the lecture series *Disease, Karma, and Healing:*

- The 'I' is stimulated by everything that repeats at 24-hour intervals.
- The soul body is stimulated by cultivating a weekly rhythm.
- The life body responds to a monthly rhythm.
- The physical body needs at least 1 year to recover fully if it has been seriously injured.

When remedies are administered to influence the regulatory activity of one constitutional member, it is recommended to incorporate the appropriate rhythm into the therapeutic model.

Constitutional treatments are not indicated in acute cases but may be administered, for example, once an illness is over or in remission. They can also be used in chronic illnesses such as allergies or diabetes to moderate the body's predisposition to disease and to work against the chronic disease process.

Therapy using homeopathic preparations of the seven main metals or certain minerals such as rubellite (red tourmaline) is central to constitutional treatment. In each instance, these therapies should be prescribed by a doctor on an individual basis and adapted to the child's constitution. Medicines suitable for self-treatment are included in the respective chapters of this book. See also the sections on Salutogenesis (page 236) and Artistic therapies (page 241).

Using specific remedies to treat imbalances or one-sided predominance in the fabric of the constitutional members is a more specifically anthroposophical form of constitutional treatment. For example, Rudolf Steiner suggests the following important remedies:

- Calcium, which restores the right balance between the physical and life bodies.
- Antimony, which brings the interaction of the life and soul bodies into rhythm.
- Quartz, which regulates the interplay of the soul body and the 'I' with healing effects on the nervous system.

Another form of anthroposophic constitutional treatment is designed to stimulate the function of specific organs and organ systems. Typical remedies of this type include:

- Cardiodoron for heart and circulation disorders.
- Hepatodoron for liver weakness.
- Cephalodoron for headaches or nervous exhaustion.

Another type of treatment relates to specific susceptibility or disease. Examples include:

- Levico comp. for frequent colds.
- Gencydo for allergies.
- Mistletoe therapies for carcinomas.

Other therapeutic approaches work to balance out the excessive one-sidedness to which we humans may succumb as we attempt to repeatedly find our balance within life's polarities. These polarities include, for example: inflammation and sclerosis, metabolic-limb functions and nerve-sensory functions, neurasthenia and hysteria. Examples of this type of treatment include:

- Hepar sulfuris, which regulates inflammatory processes, depending on the potency selected.
- Scleron, which helps in cases of premature or excessive aging processes or sclerosis.

As needed, medical approaches of this type can be accompanied by artistic therapies (see page 241), external applications (see page 293), lifestyle changes (diet, consumption of stimulants, sleep, exercise etc.). Everything we do regularly, whether in education or self-education, hobbies or work, modifies some aspect of our bodily and emotional constitution. The human constitution is changeable.

13.9 Obesity

The following examples illustrate the two scenarios involving overweight children that most frequently come to our attention.

A 2-year-old who weighs as much as a 4- to 5-year-old enjoys food, has a good appetite, drinks a lot, and has at least one parent of similar build. In this case, the paediatrician is usually the only one concerned about the child's weight, impaired mobility, possible respiratory and cardiovascular symptoms, and future health. Successful treatment depends on the parents being willing to subject themselves to a weight-loss diet and follow it consistently.

A child (usually a boy) between the ages of 10 and 13, big for his age and very overweight, is being teased in school. Because of his obesity, participation in sports is difficult, and in any case the boy has little interest in physical activity. He is becoming withdrawn and is spending more and more time alone with his computer. The first question his parents ask is whether some glandular or hormonal balance is involved. The fact that the boy is tall for his age suggests that this is not the case, and the paediatrician can usually dismiss this concern. Because such children are often sensitive, it is important to look carefully for problems and conflicts at home and in school. Psychotherapy is often indicated.

In medically uncomplicated cases of juvenile obesity, success depends on activating the child's independent will. The child may come to trust their doctor, who may be able to make a 'deal' covering the following goals:

1. Choose one favourite drink or food (something that is particularly hard to do without and that has a lot of calories), like chocolate, sugary drinks, pizza or chips. This change of habit focusing on just one task will be a good exercise of their will.

2. Take up some form of movement outside school activities, such as cycling, football, dancing, rollerblading. Swimming is not so suitable as it tends to increase the appetite too much. We would recommend basic gymnastics in a group of similarly motivated youngsters. Eurythmy or speech formation, which also help strengthen the child's soul constitution, would be even better. Drama can strengthen the constitution and give more self-confidence.

3. Agree on a (realistic) goal for weight loss over the coming week (½–1 kg, 1–2 lb) and review it weekly. If the child is sufficiently self-motivated it can help to take part in a local weight-loss programme for children and teenagers.

13.10 Preventing tooth decay

In developed countries, tooth decay appeared only with our increased consumption of refined sugar. Everything that supports tooth development during the formative period also makes teeth cavity-resistant. Because effective prevention begins in early childhood when the teeth are still developing below the surface, good collaboration between parents, children and the family dentist is important.

Tooth decay

Dental cavities develop as the result of an imbalance in demineralisation and remineralisation between the surface of the teeth and the mouth. This allows certain bacteria (especially *Streptococcus mutans*)

Influences on dental health

Positive influences
- Healthy diet
- Plenty of movement (to ensure a balanced metabolism)
- Good dental hygiene
- Suitable quantity of fluoride through drinking-water and diet
- Healthy development of teeth

Negative influences
- Increased consumption of refined sugar, sweets and soft drinks
- Poor dental hygiene
- Severe illness
- Certain medications
- Excess or deficiency of fluoride
- Hereditary predisposition

---

to make organic acids out of sugar. The acids dissolve hydroxyapatite out of the dental enamel, leading to cavities. Cavities are not a fluoride-deficiency disease.

Fluoride

Fluorides are salts formed when fluorine combines with metals, metalloids or organic components. In humans, fluoride is found in the bones and teeth and is considered one of the essential trace elements.

Blood circulation transports fluoride to the bones and teeth, where it is incorporated into the hard matter as it forms. The presence of free fluoride ions in the saliva is important for the repair (remineralisation) of dental enamel.

We now know that the primary tooth-hardening effect of fluorides sets in only when the teeth break through into the oral cavity, where they are bathed in saliva. The salivary glands secrete fluorides into the mouth, where they are incorporated into the outermost layer of dental enamel, hardening it against acids and sugary foods.

Tooth decay is almost unknown in volcanic areas, where the concentration of fluorides in drinking water is higher. In these areas, however, disorders in dental enamel formation, up to and including deformities, occur when fluoride concentrations and water consumption are especially high.

Recommendation of fluoride supplementation for children, introduced decades ago, was based on the assumption that it would contribute to the development of more cavity-resistant tooth structure. More recently, this notion has been disproved.

One interesting study has also dealt with the question of the protective effect of high fluoride content in dental enamel.[8] Shark teeth consist of pure fluorapatite and therefore contain a concentration of approximately 30,000 ppm (parts per million) of stably bound fluoride, in contrast to 1,000 ppm in human dental enamel. Shark teeth might be assumed to be largely resistant to cavities due to the fluoride solidly integrated into the enamel. Over a period of 4 weeks, the study participants carried samples of human enamel and shark enamel in their mouths. Specialised technology was used to subject the samples to conditions that were extremely conducive to tooth decay. The experiment clearly showed that shark teeth are also susceptible to cavities.

Dangers of fluoride overdose

White-speckled teeth are seen increasingly commonly today, which suggests long-term overdosing with fluoride.

Recent studies have now confirmed that excessive fluoride exposure in children leads to IQs significantly lower than the average in areas with little fluoride in the water. Excessive fluoride consumption is also known to cause toxic effects on the nervous system in adults.[9] In this context it is interesting that Rudolf Steiner spoke about the complex metabolic effect of fluoride and its neurotoxic effect on intelligence in his lecture *Introducing Anthroposophic Medicine*.

Recommendations for prevention

Mainstream recommendations

Insights into the efficacy and risks of fluoride are changing and there are differing and even contradictory recommendations in different countries and from different established bodies. Briefly summarised they are:

- Brush teeth as soon as the first milk teeth appear.
- Use toothpaste with at least 1000 ppm fluoride only once your child is old enough to spit out the toothpaste.
- From age 7 use the family toothpaste containing (1350–1500 ppm fluoride).
- Brush for about 2 minutes twice a day: once before bedtime and once at another time.
- Supervise and help children up to age 7 and ensure they spit out the toothpaste and not swallow it.

Anthroposophic dentists' recommendations

We recommend children who are breastfed and enjoy a healthy diet after weaning are monitored by the family dentist but do not receive standard fluoride supplements in the form of tablets or fluoride toothpaste. Our restraint in this regard is reinforced by studies that point out possible negative effects of too much fluoride on neurological development.

It is interesting to note that nature doles out fluorides very sparingly to breastfed babies. Breast milk contains extremely little fluoride (0.01 mg per litre as compared to 0.2 mg per litre in drinking water). In other words, the mother's body protects the baby against high levels of fluoride. Since breast milk has always been considered the ultimate food for infants, we believe that these proportions are meaningful and provide a natural standard for fluoride consumption in the first year of life.

This is why we question the validity of supplying children all over the world with fluoride in increased concentrations and in the form of compounds (like aminofluorides) that do not occur in nature. There can be no doubt about the efficacy of fluoride in saliva, but for the most part the overall impact of fluoride supplementation on the child's growing body has not been considered.

If you choose this option, of course ask your local waterworks about the fluoride content of your drinking water and pay attention to the fluoride content of foods such as salt and mineral water, which can make a big difference.

We recommend a balanced diet that largely avoids refined foods such as processed sugar and white flour and regular, good dental hygiene.

Brushing teeth

Tooth brushing, done playfully and without forcing it on your child, should be introduced as early as possible. Use a good, soft, small-headed toothbrush, even for babies.

If impatient toddlers discover crumbs (or the like) 'hopping' from tooth to tooth in their mouth, they may suddenly become interested and hold still in your arms until they have found all of them, cleaning their teeth in a playful way in the process.

Because young children like chewing on their toothbrushes and soon chew them to bits, it's a good idea to keep a second brush on hand that you use yourself for doing the actual tooth cleaning.

Young children cannot clean their own teeth effectively because they have not yet grasped the spatial relationships in their mouth. The point is to help your child lay the groundwork for good dental habits. For the same reason, it is also important for kindergartens and schools to provide opportunities for tooth brushing.

Up to about age 8, however, real tooth cleaning should be done in the evening by the parents. Use a back-and-forth motion on the chewing surfaces first, then a gentle but firm circular motion on the outside surfaces (which will also thoroughly clean the gumline) and finally a vertical brushing motion from the gum to the crown on the inside surfaces.

At least rinsing the mouth after between-meal snacks is a good idea.

Toothpastes should not contain foaming agents, which loosen the connection between the cells of mucous membranes. If you use fluoridated toothpaste, use it no more than twice a day and only once the child is capable of rinsing the toothpaste out thoroughly and no longer swallows it. Because little children enjoy eating tasty toothpaste, it is easy for them to consume excessive amounts of fluoride.

13.11 Preventing rickets

Rickets is a disturbance in bone metabolism that leads to demineralisation of the bone. Vitamin D deficiency is the most frequent cause of rickets and can result from too little vitamin D absorption from sunlight and a reduced supply from food.

Vitamin D

Vitamin D is found in fish, milk, dairy products and eggs. In a separate process, vitamin D is formed in the body itself through the action of UVB light from the sun on 7-dehydrocholesterol, which is present in the skin in sufficient amounts.

Functions of vitamin D

- Raises calcium levels in the blood.
- Increases reabsorption of calcium and phosphate in the kidneys.
- Mineralises bone by increasing calcium phosphate production.
- Inhibits release of parathyroid hormone, which triggers the release of calcium from the bones.
- Immune system regulation.

Vitamin D deficiency rickets

When children are deficient in vitamin D, calcium absorption is reduced and low amounts of minerals are available to the skeleton. This results in disturbed bone-tissue formation, growth plates not calcifying properly, and ultimately leads to bone deformities, bone fractures and inhibited growth.

Causes

- Inadequate exposure to sunlight
- Inappropriate use of sunscreen
- Low vitamin D reserves in premature infants
- Dietary vitamin D deficiency (sometimes due to a vegan diet)
- Certain medications
- Diseases associated with absorption disorders (e.g., cystic fibrosis, coeliac disease)
- Diseases of the bile ducts
- Disturbances in liver synthesis
- Chronic kidney failure

Especially at risk are

- Premature babies
- Dark-skinned children in general, but especially girls originally from Asia or Africa (due to cover-up clothing)
- Children with certain chronic diseases (see above)

Symptoms

Early signs (from age 3 months plus)

- Restlessness
- Easily startled
- Emotional distress
- Physical inactivity
- Reduced muscle tension
- Perspiration on the back of the head, hands and feet
- Restless sleep
- Immune deficiency

As the disease progresses

- Flattening of the back of the head, protruding forehead, soft spots on the back of the head
- Rachitic rosary: prominent knobs of bone at the joints of the ribs
- Flattening of the side of the chest and protrusion of the front
- Curvature of the spine while sitting up, due to slackness of muscles and ligaments
- Protrusions at the ends of bones, e.g., at the wrist joints
- Joint changes such as bow legs, knock knees, rachitic pelvis
- Changes in the teeth such as enamel defects, cavities, delayed teething
- Rachitic potbelly due to abdominal muscle weakness
- Seizures (hypocalcaemic, tetany) with muzzle-like position of the lips and paw-like position of the hands
- Constipation
- Increased susceptibility to infections

Complications

- Respiratory infections such as bronchitis or pneumonia (formerly also tuberculosis).
- Reduced lung capacity due to severe deformation of the ribcage.
- Low bone density in adolescence, associated with an increased risk of developing osteoporosis in adulthood.

- Studies have shown an association between low vitamin D intake in toddlers and later risk of developing type 1 diabetes.[10]
- Rachitic tetany can occur when calcium deficiencies in the blood become so acute that spasms may result.

Prevention
Mainstream recommendations
- Breastfed babies should by given a daily oral vitamin D supplement from birth (400–500 IU of vitamin D3).
- Formula-fed infants generally need no supplementation because every litre (quart) of commercial infant formula contains approximately 400 IU of Vitamin D3.
- Premature babies with a birth weight of less than 1,500 g (3 lb 4 oz) require 800–1,000 IU per day for the first few months.
- All children aged 6 months to 5 years should be given a daily oral vitamin D supplement.
- During childhood and adolescence, 5–15 minutes of sun exposure with exposed head, arms and legs, twice weekly from April through to September is seen as the most effective means of absorbing sufficient vitamin D. While children's sensitive skin has to be protected from the sun, sunlight is vitally important for healthy development.
- Daily, vigorous outdoor exercise to build up bone mass and improve vitamin D supply through exposure to sunlight.

Administering vitamin D
- Tablets or drops are given either straight or dissolved in a teaspoon of breast milk, tea or water. Adding the supplement to a bottle means that your baby may not get all of it.

Phytin
Phytin, a substance present in grains of all sorts but especially abundant in oats, makes part of the calcium in food insoluble so it is then eliminated in the stools.

Commercial infant formula contains no phytin and is supplemented with approximately 400–600 IU of Vitamin D3 per litre (quart).

Phytin does not harm a body that gets enough light or vitamin D. Cows' milk still contains enough absorbable calcium. Low light conditions, however, make the situation worse.

Anthroposophic perspective
In the UK from November through to March, it is difficult to achieve healthy levels of vitamin D development through the skin.

That would require exposing your baby or child's face uncovered and without sunscreen to blue sky for an average of 1 hour every day. Some winters barely offer that many sunny hours and unfortunately it isn't always possible to take advantage of them when they occur.

Doubts also exist as to whether sunlight in higher latitudes is actually capable of triggering vitamin D development from November through to February, when the angle of the light is so low ('polar winter').

Giving your baby 500 IU of vitamin D in addition to amounts ingested in food (infant formula contains added vitamin D), especially in summer, is a sure way to give more than is needed.

In recent years, scientists have been constantly adjusting the recommended dosage upwards and discovering additional factors that increase need. In other words, the definition of a healthy amount is a moving target. The concept of 'too much vitamin D', which historically revealed its effects in premature sclerosis, is now more likely to be ignored.

Our experience indicates that with a healthy diet containing adequate dairy products and with regular, year-round outdoor exercise without sunscreen or cover-up clothing, 250 IU of vitamin D supplementation is enough.

If you prefer to avoid vitamin D supplementation

Fair-skinned children with appropriately cautious parents seem to be able to develop healthily without any vitamin D supplementation, but to be on the safe side, we recommend monthly check-ins with a paediatrician once a month during the winter.

Medical treatment with a constitutional remedy that stimulates light metabolism may be helpful, for example:

- Apatite/Phosphorus comp. S, 5 drops in the morning in a bit of water or tea.
- Conchae/Quercus comp. S, 1 pea-sized portion of powder in the evening.

Additional external applications such as baths are also often prescribed as preventative measures.

Children who have dark skin or certain illnesses have greater needs, which are best discussed with your paediatrician and, in case of doubt, even determined through lab tests. We urge caution when dealing with children who are more at risk. It is essential to be especially alert and to resort to vitamin D supplementation if needed. That decision should be made by the parents in consultation with a paediatrician on an individual basis. Avoiding vitamin D supplementation is not an option for premature babies and children with certain underlying illnesses.

14. Vaccination

Why are vaccinations recommended or, in some countries, mandated by law? Because individuals should be protected from the dangers of certain infectious diseases. By promoting 'herd immunity' immunising a large part of the population the likelihood of infection declines, even for the unvaccinated.

Vaccinations are carried out because humankind feels threatened by epidemics of infectious diseases. By achieving high immunisation rates, pathogens can be eliminated regionally and eventually exterminated worldwide. Eliminating measles and polio is a stated goal of national and international health policy.

Almost all countries worldwide either recommend or require vaccination of all children against the following diseases during the first 2 years of life: tuberculosis, tetanus, whooping cough, diphtheria, polio, Hib (Haemophilus Influenzae), hepatitis B, pneumococcal, measles, mumps and rubella (German measles) and meningitis. These recommendations continually change, and as well as variations between different countries, there are variations between states within some countries.

Parents should find out about the latest recommendations locally: if unsure, ask your doctor.

On the way to achieving these goals, however, a number of problems, still unresolved, have been encountered. Wherever laws permit parents to decide which immunisations their children should receive, the risks and benefits of currently recommended inoculations should be openly debated, along with their possible indirect effects on the development of immunity. Ideally, parents (in consultation with their doctors) should be free to decide whether and when their children will be vaccinated and which vaccines they will receive.

We hope to provide our readers with a basis for making sound decisions on these serious issues. If you have read Sections 15.3–15.4 on the meaning and ethical aspects of illness, you will not be surprised to find that our approach to vaccination is quite different from what is usually found in books of medical advice. We hope our approach will help parents make decisions that take into account both their child's individual situation and the long-term good of society. We assume, however, that parents who avoid indiscriminate vaccination will be able to provide their children with the necessary rest, treatment and convalescence if the illnesses in question do appear. This includes avoiding travelling with a sick child and allowing adequate time for recovery.

14.1 What do vaccinations do?

The purpose of vaccinations is to prevent specific infectious diseases. Vaccines (administered orally, by injection or by scratching them into the skin) stimulate the body to produce protective substances identical or similar to the 'antibodies' that develop when the body overcomes an infectious disease. The resulting immunity confers varying degrees of protection from the illness for periods of time that may also vary among individuals. Vaccination is thus a form of artificial immunisation.

There are two types of immunisation: active and passive.

Active immunisation

Active immunisation can be subdivided into two types:
• 'Live' vaccines containing attenuated pathogens (which have been weakened but are still capable of reproduction).

• 'Dead' vaccines produced from killed pathogens or their breakdown or metabolic products.

Active immunisation confers immunity for years, sometimes lifelong with live vaccines.

Passive immunisation

Passive immunisation gives antibodies that protect against particular acute diseases. Because these foreign antibodies break down rapidly in the body, passive immunisation confers effective protection for a few months at most.

Possible drawbacks for the immune system

Because the standard recommendation is to administer most vaccines during the first year of life, vaccinations typically occur when both the immune system and the nervous system are most actively developing.

It is difficult to either prove or disprove whether vaccinations change the immune system in ways that favour the development of allergies or autoimmune disorders, and mandatory studies conducted prior to the introduction of vaccines certainly do not address this possibility. One example of a possible questionable effect on the immune system is the as yet unexplained increase in juvenile diabetes in industrialised nations.

Because allergies and auto-immune disorders appear only much later and studies are usually designed to cover periods of three years or less, few definitive findings on possible negative impacts of immunisation are available to date. However, studies that have explicitly investigated the connection between vaccinations and allergies tended to find increases in allergic problems.

Thus the question of possible excessive demands on the immune system due to the ever-increasing number of components of multiple vaccines must indeed be taken seriously and is not conclusively answered by the statement that all of these vaccines are safe and effective.

Possible side effects of vaccinations
Minor reactions
- Headache
- Fever
- Local reddening, swelling
- Tiredness
- Crankiness

Severe reactions
- Cramps
- Abscesses
- Allergic reactions, even allergic (anaphylactic) shock
- Apathy, over-excitability, shrill crying
- Breathing arrest in infants

Complications
Occasionally, chronic or permanent effects can occur following vaccination. These include:
- Neuritis
- Meningitis
- Encephalitis
- Guillain–Barré syndrome
- Further autoimmune diseases are suspected, like multiple sclerosis, type 1 diabetes, rheumatism and the increase in allergic sensitivities and autism.
- Vaccine-induced illness can occur after vaccination with live vaccines. The disease the vaccine is designed to prevent manifests in a weakened form, as in vaccine-induced measles.

A list of rare and debatable side effects associated with specific vaccines can be found in the section on each vaccine.

14.2 Making individual choices

In many Western countries, parents are completely free to decide for or against vaccinating their children and therefore also bear the greatest responsibility. The government, or its panel of experts, simply issues public recommendations. It is essential for the parents and the consulting doctor, who may also be the one who would administer the vaccine, to take the child's individual situation and social integration into account.

Parents with reservations about vaccinations usually consult a doctor with a homeopathic, naturopathic or anthroposophic orientation.

Individual consultations

In informative sessions with the parents, the doctor first tries to be responsive to the parents' ideas, to clear away biases and misinformation, to introduce fundamental aspects that broaden the perspective and to avoid exerting moral pressure. The next step is to come to an individually appropriate decision regarding immunisation.

Topics of discussion include the spacing of immunisations, available combination vaccines and possible complications, as well as any vaccines that may be contraindicated for the child in question. In cases of severe congenital or acquired heart or lung disease or other illnesses and syndromes, the vaccines that are important and possible in such cases are pointed out to the parents.

Possible disadvantages of early vaccination are considered with respect to the development of the immune and nervous systems.

Individual risks related to the child's health and living situation and the family's travel habits and contacts are discussed. Alternative immunisation schedules from other countries are also mentioned.

In Norway, for example, immunisations begin only at 3 months with a pentavalent vaccine plus pneumococcus. Instead of 3 additional doses, only 2 are given, at 5 and 12 months. Also, hepatitis B, chickenpox and rotavirus immunisations are not part of the standard package. Clearly, therefore, the recommendations and decisions of experts in comparable situations can differ.

As a result of our consultations with parents, we frequently vaccinate later (often when the child is walking) and against significantly fewer diseases than government recommendations. This approach requires thoroughly educating the parents in advance about the diseases and their risks.

Additional perspectives and positions can be found in the sections on individual vaccines (see below).

14.3 Tetanus

The illness

Tetanus is rare in affluent countries, but is more common in tropical countries with a low tetanus vaccination rate and has a higher mortality rate, particularly among babies of unvaccinated mothers. It is a serious illness involving muscle spasms. It is fatal in 30–50% of cases in adults who contract the infection.

The tetanus germ is the bacterium *Clostridium tetani*. It is capable of forming spores and is very resistant to outer influences, such as antiseptics and heat. The spores are found in the earth, often in horse or cattle dung, and rarely in other animal excrements. The bacteria grow best in oxygen-free environments where they can form the tetanus toxin.

The vaccination

In USA and the UK, the officially recommended schedule of vaccinations includes 3 tetanus vaccinations administered in combination with diphtheria and whooping cough (pertussis) as DTP vaccine, or with others in the 6-in-1 vaccine, given 3 times at ages 8 weeks, 12 weeks and 16 weeks. In the UK, it is also included in the 4-in-1 preschool booster given at age 3 years, and the 3-in-1 teenage booster, given at 13 years.

We think it makes sense to vaccinate healthy children only once they are walking, when their neurological and immunological development is more advanced. In addition, if the mother has been vaccinated, the relevant antibodies are transmitted to the baby during pregnancy and provide protection that lasts for months. As there is no single diphtheria vaccination, a decision about tetanus vaccination has to be made together with that of diphtheria.

Vaccination after injury

Tetanus bacteria can enter your skin through cuts and grazes, animal bites and burns, for example. One-time booster shots of vaccine can be administered after injuries occurring more than 5 years after the last vaccination, or even earlier if the wound is very dirty or if the patient has severe injuries, especially burns.

With children, a parent's attention quickly soothes the pain of minor abrasions. Gentle cleansing with lukewarm tap water, followed by exposure to air and light, is enough to ensure proper healing. A risk of tetanus infection exists only in deeper, dirty wounds with no exposure to oxygen in the air.

14.4 Diphtheria

The illness

The diphtheria pathogen is the bacterium *Corynebacterium diphtheria*. For the disease to manifest, formation of the diphtheria toxin must occur. In temperate climatic zones, most diphtheria cases tend to peak in autumn and winter. In Western industrialised countries, incidence of diphtheria has declined considerably, but although a decrease has also been observed in other parts of the world, regional outbreaks still occur.

For information on the symptoms and course of the illness, see page 148.

In Europe in recent years, diphtheria-like infections with the toxigenic *Corynebakterium ulcerans* have been observed more frequently than illnesses due to the actual diphtheria pathogen. The diphtheria vaccine is assumed but has not been proven to be effective against these germs. There have been isolated cases in Germany where at least a few of the patients had been routinely vaccinated.

The vaccination

In USA and the UK, officially recommended diphtheria immunisation, like tetanus immunisation, is included in the 6-in-1 vaccine, given 3 times at ages 8 weeks, 12 weeks and 16 weeks. In the UK, it is also included in the 4-in-1 preschool booster given at age 3 years, and the 3-in-1 teenage booster, given at 13 years.

For reasons discussed above in the section on tetanus vaccination, we recommend that when diphtheria vaccination is desired, parents should postpone the vaccination until the child is a year old, unless there are concerns about a possible epidemic or when travelling in areas of higher risk.

14.5 Haemophilus influenzae type B bacteria (Hib)

The illness

Haemophilus influenzae type B bacteria (Hib) are involved in cases of acute life-threatening epiglottitis (see page 71) and, before vaccination was possible, often in purulent meningitis and middle-ear infections in childhood.

The germs are also found in approximately 5% of healthy children. The bacteria is difficult to detect and can cause severe infections, including meningitis and acute epiglottitis. Before the vaccine became available, approximately 1 infant in 500 experienced a serious Hib infection. This means that the others developed immunity with no signs of illness.

The risk is greater in low-income populations and highest in children with congenital or illness-induced immunodeficiencies and in individuals with no spleen or minimal spleen function.

The vaccination

The current recommendation in USA and the UK is to give the 6-in-1 vaccine, given 3 times at ages 8 weeks, 12 weeks and 16 weeks. In the UK, a Hib vaccination is also given when the child is 1 year old, in combination with a Men C vaccine.

Contrary to popular belief, Hib vaccination does not offer universal protection against meningitis but only against one of several meningitis germs. Since the introduction of the vaccine, infection rates have declined rapidly, as have the occasional initially reported cases of vaccine failure. Clearly, immunisation efforts have retarded the circulation of the germ.

14.6 Whooping cough (pertussis)

The illness

The pertussis pathogen is *Bordetella pertussis*, a small, immobile, encapsulated bacterium. It multiplies on the bronchial mucous membranes and produces certain toxins that cause tissue damage. It can appear at any time of year, but in Central Europe the highest incidence is observed in autumn and winter.

For information on the symptoms and course of the illness, see page 145.

The vaccination

The current recommendation in USA and the UK is to give the 6-in-1 vaccine, given 3 times at ages 8 weeks, 12 weeks and 16 weeks. In the UK, it is also included in the 4-in-1 preschool booster given at age 3 years.

There are potential problems with this vaccine. As an example, a study conducted in Australia during a whooping cough epidemic from December 2008 revealed that fully immunised 2- to 3-year-old siblings were the most (and increasingly) frequent source of infection for infants under 6 months, due to the immune system's poor response to whooping cough vaccinations. The failure rate of vaccines is 30–50%, with an additional 20–25% of those vaccinated experiencing a milder course of the disease.

The following considerations reveal the difficulties facing any meaningful vaccination strategy, especially in the case of whooping cough.

Cocoon strategy

In this scenario, people in contact with the child, such as parents, grandparents, childcare providers etc., are vaccinated. People in close contact with infants, primarily their mothers, are responsible for ⅓–⅔ of pertussis (whooping cough) cases in young infants. However, more than 5,000 contact persons would have to be vaccinated to prevent a single case of whooping cough in an infant, 10,000 to prevent a hospitalisation, and 1 million to prevent a single fatality. Herd immunity is unreliable, because even vaccinated individuals can carry and excrete pertussis bacteria.[11]

Vaccination during pregnancy (after week 30)

Transplacental transmission of whooping cough antibodies could protect the infant against coincidental exposure to whooping cough, which is responsible for approximately ⅓ of infections.[12] This strategy is cheaper and more effective than the cocoon strategy, but its safety for the unborn baby has not yet been confirmed.

Vaccinating newborns

It is true that the incidence of whooping cough in childhood initially decreased in heavily immunised populations. This strategy has gaps, however. There are enough examples of children who have been vaccinated 3 or 4 times but still contract whooping cough around age 5.

The groups that the vaccine is actually intended to protect are: some children with chronic illnesses, premature babies and infants up to the age of 6 months. The two latter groups are not yet fully protected by early vaccination, and the recommended strategy aims instead to reduce opportunities for older siblings and parents to infect infants.

Another disadvantage is that the body responds with lower antibody levels when a child is later vaccinated against whooping cough, Hib and hepatitis B.

A different problem is that in spite of high vaccination rates, eliminating the disease can be hindered not only directly, through vaccination failure, but also by the fact that viruses may survive in non-human hosts (e.g. animals) and then produce further outbreaks when immunity lapses or if vaccination was not successful in the first place.

The higher the vaccination rates, the more adults become sources of infections for little babies. Adults usually experience only a nagging cough that lingers for several weeks and are contagious without ever realising they have whooping cough. Stepping up the immunisation strategy would do at least a somewhat better job of reaching these adults. Increasingly, however, it is children who have been vaccinated but not effectively immunised or who have experienced a mild course of the illness who pose an unrecognised and unpredictable risk for their little siblings (see above).

In our experience, a parent's availability during the illness plays a decisive and positive role, especially for very young children. Here, presence is the best means of relieving fear of suffocation, which significantly intensifies the bouts of coughing.

Vaccination makes sense for patients with certain lung and heart diseases and in certain social situations, such as refugee camps or crowded dwellings with large numbers of children.

For the dangers associated with whooping cough in infants, see page 145.

14.7 Polio

The illness
The cause of polio, or infantile paralysis, is the poliovirus. Vaccination efforts since the 1950s have virtually eliminated polio, with only Afghanistan and Pakistan having endemic outbreaks in the last 3 years.

Polio is transmitted primarily by smear infection via the faecal–oral route, with an incubation period of anywhere from 3–35 days. Over 95% of cases are asymptomatic, and flu-like symptoms without involvement of the central nervous system occur in approximately 4%. In 1% of cases, the central nervous system is infected, resulting in symptoms such as muscle stiffness, muscle pain and paralysis. The paralysis may be permanent and may also affect the respiratory and muscular systems. Fatalities have been known to occur. There is no specific treatment.

The vaccination
In the USA and UK, the polio vaccination is given in the 6-in-1 vaccine, given 3 times at ages 8

weeks, 12 weeks and 16 weeks. In the UK, it is also included in the 4-in-1 preschool booster given at age 3 years, and the 3-in-1 teenage booster, given at 13 years.

As an alternative, for example, before travelling to an area where polio is still active, 2 doses of inactivated polio virus (IPV) separated by 8 weeks to 6 months are adequate. Europe has been free of wild polio infections for a number of years. The individual risk of contracting the disease has become minimal, and the WHO goal of eradicating polio worldwide in just a few years once seemed realistic. Recent discoveries of circulating mutated viruses derived from oral vaccines in poor countries, however, are reducing this hope.

For adolescents and adults, an IPV booster shot is recommended only before travelling to countries where there is a risk of contracting polio.

14.8 Chickenpox (varicella)

The illness
Chickenpox is caused by the *Varicella zoster* virus. As a rule, the course of the illness is mild and patients recover without complications. For further details, see page 140.

The vaccination
In the UK, the chickenpox vaccine is available in addition to the routine vaccination programme to 'at risk' babies and children, for example siblings of children whose immune systems are suppressed (e.g. because they have had an organ transplant) and are susceptible to chickenpox. The vaccine can be given to children aged 1 year and over. Two doses of the vaccine are given 4–8 weeks apart.

As a result of routine vaccination of children against chickenpox in other parts of the world, for example the USA, the disease has been appearing in other age groups at risk of further complications. Moreover, increased cases of shingles are to be expected. And since chickenpox can be seen as a harmless childhood illness (for possible complications, see page 141), we do not recommend vaccination for healthy children without either an immunodeficiency syndrome or a severe tendency to eczema.

14.9 Rubella (German measles)

The illness
The rubella pathogen is the rubella virus. The infection it causes is

generally harmless but can have fatal consequences if women contract it for the first time during pregnancy. For them, it is a huge emotional burden to be infected with rubella and learn that they have no antibodies.

The risk of miscarriage from rubella in the first 11 weeks of pregnancy is as high as 90%, and defects (especially of the inner ear) can still be expected in up to 5% of babies when the infection occurs after week 16 of pregnancy. Possible delayed consequences include diabetes and the development of autism.

For further details, see page 132.

The vaccination

In the UK, a vaccine for rubella is included in the MMR vaccine (measles, mumps and rubella). It is given when the child is 1 year old and again at 3 years and 4 months.

Since 1973, an injectable live vaccine against rubella has been officially recommended. Its only purpose is preemptive immunisation of girls to prevent damage to unborn children in the future.

This policy, however, is not optimal. From the epidemiological perspective, the vaccine should be administered only to girls in puberty to avoid disrupting the acquisition of immunity through natural means. Meanwhile we know from experience that widespread vaccination of women of childbearing age results in lower levels of antibodies in vaccinated women than in unvaccinated people, assuming that the latter have developed immunity through infection or contact with the wild virus.

Even if their concentration of antibodies is lower, unvaccinated women are much less likely to contract rubella for the second time during pregnancy than vaccinated women are. Repeated vaccinations are also less effective than being infected with the wild virus.

14.10 Mumps

The illness

The mumps pathogen is a virus belonging to the family of paramyxoviruses. As a childhood illness, mumps is generally harmless, with severe cases being more common in adults.

Nowadays, almost all children recover from mumps meningitis (meningoencephalitis) without lasting damage (see page 143), and the symptoms are not severe enough to be used as the chief argument in support of vaccination. The only possible remaining motive for vaccination is to prevent permanent damage such as rare (and fortunately usually one-sided) hearing loss.

It is now known that inflammation of the testes, a rare but possible complication of mumps, does not necessarily lead to male infertility, as was previously assumed. Once again, it is quite difficult to assess actual risks of testicular inflammation with or without vaccination.

The current state of our knowledge, with the exception of epidemic differences in severity and susceptibility, suggests taking the following approach to mumps vaccination.

Let's suppose that parents are wondering whether or not to have their 18-month-old son vaccinated. Prior to the introduction of the vaccine, most children contracted mumps before the age of 15. 70–90% of adults today developed antibodies through either infection or exposure prior to the era of immunisation. Assuming that the boy does not grow up to be one of these adults but remains susceptible to mumps into adulthood, the question remains whether he would develop silent immunity or a symptomatic infection as a result of exposure to the wild virus. If he does contract the disease later in life, his chances of developing one-sided testicular inflammation are 20–30%. At the moment, even doctors cannot provide more precise information.

People need to be aware of this state of affairs because the simple statement that 'mumps can cause testicular inflammation with permanent infertility' is not a very accurate characterisation of the actual risk.

Permanent inner-ear damage is also one-sided in most cases. Because it is often diagnosed only much later, incidence figures are unreliable, but in general we can expect roughly 1 case of serious hearing loss for every 15,000 cases of uncomplicated mumps. In 30 years of practising paediatrics, we have met only 1 child with mumps-related hearing loss. But as vaccination becomes more common, we must expect the age of peak susceptibility among unvaccinated individuals to increase, and complications are more frequent in adults.

Mumps encephalitis (see page 141), which can cause lasting damage to the brain or nerves, is a rare complication of mumps. This must not to be confused with mumps meningitis/meningoencephalitis (see page 143), a common and usually harmless complication of mumps. Sources disagree about its incidence. Mumps encephalitis is reported to cause less severe symptoms than measles encephalitis. We have never seen a patient with mumps encephalitis.

The vaccination

In the UK, a vaccine for mumps is included in the MMR vaccine (measles, mumps and rubella). It is given when the child is 1 year old and again at 3 years and 4 months. Mumps vaccination as part of the MMR vaccine is officially recommended in most developed countries.

It is not known how long immunity due to vaccination lasts, but is assumed to be about 10–15 years. The current vaccination strategy will certainly not achieve the high degree of immunity formerly common among adults. There is a danger of epidemics among adolescents and adults with increased risks of complications.

The vaccination is useful for men. As the immunity does not last into adulthood, we believe that delaying vaccination for boys until puberty is appropriate, though this must be considered together with measles and rubella, as it is a combination vaccine.

14.11 Measles

The illness

The measles pathogen is a virus belonging to the family of paramyxoviruses. This germ is extremely contagious. Measles can occur anywhere in the world but can be found in Africa in particular. Measles is one of the ten most common infectious diseases, and the percentage of fatal outcomes is especially high.

For further details, see page 128.

The vaccination

In the UK, a vaccine for measles is included in the MMR vaccine (measles, mumps and rubella). It is given when the child is 1 year old and again at 3 years and 4 months.

Vaccine-induced measles are a possibility, generally developing 7–12 days after vaccination and accompanied by fever and perhaps any of the other symptoms of measles. This is assumed to be a sign that the first vaccination was successful, and antibody detection supports this, but it does not reflect the more effective form of resistance. After the first vaccination about 93% have resistance. The second vaccination has no effect on the 93%, but increases the overall protection to about 95%.

Protective vaccination against measles can also be administered up to 3 days after exposure, since immunity develops more rapidly after vaccination than symptoms can appear (see also page 128). This prophylactic vaccination is not on the official list of universally recommended vaccines, but it may be indicated in certain situations.

It is well known that in free and democratic countries willingness to accept vaccination actually declines among the general population when pro-vaccination propaganda peaks. Hence health authorities must realise that they will be able to eliminate measles only through measures such as legally required isolation of patients and mandatory vaccination. But where the proportion of unvaccinated to vaccinated individuals is similar to what it is in Germany, for example, failure to isolate cases of infection offers vaccinated individuals repeated opportunities for additional immunity, while preserving freedom of choice with regard to vaccination.

We must emphasise, however, that a measles epidemic may cause a few fatalities.

If your child is not vaccinated and has not had measles by the time they are 9–12 years old, we recommend revisiting the question of immunisation, because the risk of complications increases with puberty. Measles in the first year of life is a more recent problem. The passive immunity transmitted by mothers who were immunised as children may not be sufficient to protect their infants. New observations show that the dreaded panencephalitis (SSPE), at an incidence of 1 in 5000, is much more common when measles occurs in infancy than if the disease is contracted later. You may choose to have your own child vaccinated because they might infect and endanger an infant.

There is also an important emotional consequence of vaccination that remains to be considered. Parents who have their children vaccinated against as many contagious diseases as possible, including measles, are as a rule more afraid of these and other illnesses than parents who do not. We have seen instances in which vaccinated kindergarten children were not allowed to ride in the same car with unvaccinated youngsters, in spite of the fact that exposure to the wild virus would have enhanced the limited immunity conferred by vaccination. Even in cases of vaccine failure, an outbreak of measles in vaccinated children is much less dangerous at this age than it is later.

14.12 Rotavirus vaccination

The illness

Rotaviruses are the most common cause of viral intestinal infections in childhood. Children between the ages of 6 months and 2 years are the most commonly affected. Transmission is by smear infection (direct contact with an infected person, or touching a contaminated object). The incubation period is 1–3 days.

In infections accompanied by diarrhoea, rotaviruses can be excreted in the stools for up to 14 days. Thorough hygiene such as washing the hands with soap helps to prevent transmission.

The main symptoms are vomiting and diarrhoea (yellow-green and foul-smelling), often accompanied by fever. There is the danger of dehydration in young infants. In severe cases hospitalisation is required so that fluids can be administered intravenously, but in most cases treatment with a bland diet and electrolyte solutions to drink is sufficient.

Breastfed infants are less likely to develop diarrhoea.

Life-threatening cases are uncommon, occurring primarily in children with specific risk factors such as a serious primary disease or extreme prematurity.

Timely hospitalisation is important in order to avoid fatalities.

For warning symptoms that require immediate hospitalisation, see page 87.

Diarrhoeal illnesses are a major problem in developing countries, where they contribute to high child mortality.

The vaccination

In the UK, the rotavirus vaccine is given orally to babies at 8 weeks and 12 weeks. The vaccine protects against severe rotavirus infections and is intended to prevent hospitalisations due to the illness.

Children can contract rotavirus infections in spite of having been vaccinated, but as a rule the illness is less severe in those cases.

Breastfeeding significantly reduces the risk of illness because antibodies present in breast milk target the rotaviruses. Thus it is recommended to avoid nursing for 1 hour before and 1 hour after vaccination, if your baby's rhythm permits, in order to get the best results from the vaccine.

Side effects

In addition to frequent gastrointestinal symptoms such as vomiting and diarrhoea, the vaccine can lead to intussception, meaning that the bowel folds into itself. In the worst case scenario, bowel blockage or perforation can develop. Intussception is a typical complication of rotavirus, whether wild or in the form of vaccine.

While vaccination does reduce the risk of illness, intussceptions increase. The rate in the UK is currently about 2 in every 100,000 babies vaccinated.

We recommend a thorough consideration of the possible risks and benefits. In our view, breastfed children with no risk factors have sufficient immune competence to get through the illness without severe symptoms.

14.13 Respiratory syncytial virus (RSV)

The illness

The respiratory syncytial virus (RSV) is considered one of the most frequent causes of upper and lower respiratory infections in children. It is spread by droplet infection. Cases peak during the winter.

Cases with severe bronchitis or pneumonia can occur in infants, often requiring intensive care and oxygen administration, sometimes in conjunction with a breathing aid or mechanical ventilation.

Symptoms
- Rhinitis
- Cough
- Fever
- Shortness of breath
- Problems with drinking

Risk groups
High risk
- Babies born before week 29 of pregnancy.
- Children who have been treated with oxygen for lung disease in late autumn/early winter (peak RSV season is October to March).
- Children with serious heart defects.

Moderate risk
- Premature babies born after week 29 of gestation and discharged from the hospital during winter.
- Children with severe neurological disorders.
- Children cared for outside of the family during the first year of life.

Immunisation

In this case, there is no widely available vaccine. However, in the UK, antibodies against RSV are available for children with a high risk of contracting the infection, and can be considered for those at medium risk. These are administered monthly via intramuscular injection during wintertime. The effect begins with the first dose, but maximum efficacy is achieved only after the second dose. These antibodies reduce the risk of a hospital admission, but complications or fatalities cannot be ruled out.

14.14 Tuberculosis (BCG vaccine)

The illness
Tuberculosis is a bacterial infection that is spread through inhaling droplets from an infected person's coughs and sneezes. The pathogen is *Mycobacterium tuberculosis*. The lungs are most frequently affected. Tuberculosis occurs worldwide.

Vaccination and prevention

In the UK, vaccination has not been officially recommended since 2005 due to its inadequate efficacy. In North America, it is recommended only where there is a special risk of infection. In Ireland and South Africa, the BCG (Bacille Calmette Suerin) vaccine is administered at birth.

Tuberculosis vaccination does not offer reliable protection against infection or illness, nor does it (as is repeatedly claimed) lessen the severity of symptoms. More important are:
- Diagnosing, treating and supervising actively tubercular patients.
- Ensuring that TB patients do not infect small children.
- Vaccinating cows and pasteurising milk from farms that cannot be reliably certified as TB-free.

Tuberculin tests yield positive results in both vaccinated and infected individuals, so vaccine failures (infections that occur in spite of vaccination) are more difficult to identify in vaccinated populations. Newborns must be protected from infection by isolating them from suspected actively tubercular patients.

14.15 Hepatitis A

The illness
The hepatitis pathogen is the hepatitis A virus (HAV). Transmission is by smear infection, via the faecal–oral route. The virus is present worldwide. In developing countries, almost all individuals contract the infection in childhood or adolescence. People from countries with high standards of hygiene have very low immunity, so they are at risk of HAV infec-

tion when they travel to countries where the disease is prevalent.

For further details, see page 150.

The vaccination

In the UK, a vaccine for hepatitis A is not routinely recommended because of the low risk of infection. Usually it is recommended only for people at high risk, including people in contact with someone who already has hepatitis A, people with long-term liver conditions, or people travelling to countries where the risk of infection is high. Vaccination is often recommended for children if they are travelling to high-risk areas. Vaccinations should be given 2–3 weeks before travel, and can be repeated after 6–12 months to give long-term protection. Alternatively, follow the general rule: 'Peel it, cook it or leave it.'

Jaundice is symptom of hepatitis A, so when cases of jaundice appear in schools or kindergartens, vaccination with active hepatitis A vaccine (HAV) is recommended for the children who are not yet ill. Since hepatitis A infections are almost always mild in children, we recommend thorough bathroom hygiene and case-by-case decisions on whether or not to vaccinate.

14.16 Hepatitis B

The illness

The hepatitis B virus is the hepatitis B pathogen. The illness, a liver infection, is one of the most common infectious diseases. Transmission occurs primarily through blood or vaginal or sperm secretions.

For further information, see page 151.

The vaccination

In North America and South Africa, hepatitis B vaccination is universally recommended for infants. In the USA, the vaccine is given in 3 doses: at birth, at 1–2 months, and finally at 6–18 months. Older children and adolescents can get a catch-up vaccination. In South Africa, the vaccine is given in 4 doses: within 7 days of birth, and at 6 weeks, 4 months and 6 months. The reasons for this recommendation are increases in prevalence of the virus among teenagers and adults and the presence of chronic contagious cases in the general population.

However, in the UK the vaccination is not routinely administered. It is only recommended for babies born to mothers infected with hepatitis B, and to children at high risk of exposure to the virus. If required, it will be given in

6 doses: at birth, then at 4, 8, 12 and 16 weeks, with the final dose at 1 year old.

The risk of infection in infants in the Western world is extremely low. Of course we provide passive and active vaccination when needed to protect an infant whose mother has contagious hepatitis B. In general, we restrict our use of the vaccine in infants and older children to cases of high risk.

14.17 Pneumococcal vaccination

The illness

Worldwide, pneumococci (*Streptococcus pneumoniae*) are among the most common causes of inflammations of the lungs, meninges, middle ear and sinuses. Transmission occurs via droplet infection. There are over 90 different known groups of pneumococci, varyingly distributed throughout the world. Immunocompromised individuals are especially at risk. Protective measures include, among others, breastfeeding and avoiding smoking in the presence of children. Antibiotic treatment is indicated when a pneumococcus infection occurs.

The vaccination

In the UK, the pnemococcal (or pneumo) inoculation is a routine vaccination given at 8 weeks, 16 weeks and 1 year old.

The pneumococci are a very large group of closely related bacteria (serogroups), which means that any vaccine needs to contain antigens from different serogroups. It should be noted that the prevalence of different strains of pneumococci often varies from country to country. The vaccine that is currently used in USA contains antigens from 7 (out of more than 40 possible) serogroups and was developed for that country, so it is not fine-tuned to pneumococcal strains in other countries. As a result, it may not offer reliable protection against suppurative meningitis.

We recommend that this vaccine is used only for 'children at risk', extremely premature births and children who fail to thrive or have severe underlying illnesses.

14.18 Meningococcal vaccinations

The illness

Meningococci (*Neisseria meningitidis*) are bacteria that can trigger a variety of syndromes. Approximately 10% of the population carry these bacteria in their nasal cavity but are asymptomatic. The infection is carried on droplets and transmitted from person to person during coughing, sneezing or kissing. If the immune system is weakened, meningitis or sepsis (blood poisoning) with internal bleeding may develop, sometimes becoming life-threatening within hours, which require intensive hospital care and antibiotic treatment.

For further details on meningitis, see page 27.

The vaccination

Since 2006, most Western countries have recommended meningococcal vaccination. In the UK, there are two separate vaccinations for meningococci: the Men B vaccine and the Men C vaccine (the latter in combination with the Hib vaccine). The Men B vaccine protects against meningitis caused by the meningococcal type B bacteria, and is given in 3 doses, at 8 weeks, 16 weeks and 1 year old. The Hib/Men C vaccine protects against Hib (see page 265) and meningitis caused by the meningococcal group C bacteria, and is given in 1 dose at 1 year old.

The Men C vaccine consists of inactivated meningococcal bacteria and is administered once. Duration of protection is relatively short: toddlers for about a year, older children and adolescents up to 5 years.

The most common side effect is a fever 3 days after the vaccination. There have also been some reported cases of Kawasaki disease that affects the blood vessels and can harm the coronary arteries. We do not recommend these vaccinations except for children who are at risk due to immunodeficiency or for travel to high-risk countries.

14.19 Human papilloma virus (HPV)

The illness

Worldwide, HPV is the most common sexually transmitted virus. Of the more than 100 different types of HPV, over 35 affect the female genital tract and 25 are currently considered carcinogenic. HPV is found in 1 out of every 3 women within 24 months of first sexual contact, and over 70% of all women will become infected with one of the different types of HPV in the course of their lives.

HPV infection is usually asymptomatic and resolves spontaneously within 1–2 years in 90% of cases. The younger the woman at the time of infection, the greater the probability of this natural healing.

After 1 year, HPV can no longer be detected in 80% of those affected. Reinfection is unlikely once a woman has had one HPV infection.

Because genetic material from human papilloma viruses can be detected in women with cervical cancer, a causal relationship is assumed, but the development of cancer is more dependent on the woman's individual susceptibility than on infection. Years to decades can elapse between permanent implantation of the virus and the development of changes in the mucosal cells. Because smear tests permit very early detection of cervical cancer, the greatest importance must be placed on routine, preventative gynaecological exams for adult women.

The vaccination

Since about 2007 authorities have been recommending immunisation against the human papilloma virus (HPV) for all girls between the ages of 11 and 15 prior to first sexual intercourse. In the UK, girls from age 12–18 can get the HPV vaccine, which is given in 2 doses: the first is from age 12–13 years, and the second follows 6–12 months later.

The duration of protection is not yet clear, so that infection may occur at a later age when natural healing declines. There are recent reports of strong side effects in young women, such as chronic pain, fatigue and circulation problems. We recommend a thorough consideration of the possible risks and benefits.

The vaccination is definitely no substitute for routine cervical screening, which will also detect cancer.

14.20 Flu (influenza)

The illness

The flu is caused by the influenza virus, of which there are different types: A, B and C. Transmission is by droplet infection. The disease is highly contagious and the incubation period is short. For further information, see page 66. Serious flu epidemics seem to appear almost every winter. These epidemics are triggered by a highly variable group of viruses.

The vaccination

In the UK, the flu vaccine is offered to children from age 6 months up to 17 years, though eligibility differs depending on which area of the UK you live in. Check with your doctor to see if your child is entitled to the vaccination.

Because of the highly variable group of viruses, vaccines (made of isolated antigens) must be reformulated each year according to which type of virus appears. There is always a degree of uncertainty as to whether the new vaccine contains the appropriate antigens. The independent research group Cochrane has evaluated the published results of the effectiveness of the flu vaccine as unproven.

We recommend flu vaccinations only for high-risk patients and for age groups or professional groups that face exceptional risks.

14.21 Tick-borne encephalitis

The illness

Spring-summer meningoencephalitis (also called tick-borne or Central European encephalitis, not to be confused with Lyme disease, see page 152) is an infection carried by ticks. It occurs in a broad band from Central Europe to East Asia.

The vaccination

Tick-borne encephalitis is not found in the UK, but there is a low risk of contracting it if travelling in parts of Europe and Asia. Vaccinations can be obtained for a cost at private travel clinics in the UK. Effective protection requires an initial vaccination 1 month before travelling followed by two others (2 weeks to 3 months later, and 9–12 months later) or, on an accelerated schedule, an initial vaccination followed by second and third shots 7 and 21 days later with a booster 1 year later. Boosters are recommended every 3 years for those who spend long periods of time in areas of risk.

Active vaccination is recommended for agricultural and forestry workers and for people travelling or taking part in recreational sports in areas of known risk.

Because the disease is generally milder in children and seldom causes permanent damage, and because often feverish and occasionally neurological reactions have been observed in vaccinated babies and toddlers, this vaccine is not recommended for children under age 3.

Passive vaccination is not possible after being bitten by ticks. Tick bites can be largely prevented by wearing clothing that covers the entire body and by applying natural insect repellents (such as carnation oil/Aetheroleum caryophylli). In South Africa, Tick Safe is an available product. These measures offer simultaneous protection against tick-borne Lyme disease (see page 152), a disease that cannot be prevented by vaccination and is often very serious.

15. Facing Tough Challenges

15.1 Being admitted to hospital

Accompanying a child

The younger the children, the more essential it is for them to be accompanied by a parent or other trusted adult when they are admitted to hospital. For this reason, many hospitals now accommodate parents who wish to spend the night with their child. Where special accommodation is not available, parents should do everything they can to ensure that one of them is allowed to stay with the child. For preschool children, the constant presence of a parent should be seen as an essential part of medical care. We sincerely hope that in future all paediatric wards will be designed to allow parents to stay with their children.

While illness removes children from their accustomed daily routine, hospitalisation also tears them away from familiar surroundings. Under these unusual circumstances, all impressions have a greater than normal impact on a child's soul. The greatest possible love and attention are needed to ensure that hospitalisation is not a damaging experience. Doctors, nurses and parents should do everything they can to ensure that children have positive memories of periods in hospital. If children have parents with them, that familiar continuity can compensate for the bewildering new surroundings.

When a parent cannot (or, in the case of an older child, need not) be admitted along with the child, flexible visiting hours are essential so that children can see their closest relatives at any time.

When children are hospitalised for longer periods, it is important to provide stimuli for age-appropriate play and learning. Hospitals do not always have occupational therapists available, or a play group or hospital classes, so parents need to take the initiative here.

Talking about illness

Adults need to be sensitive to whether (and when) children

hospitalised with serious or life-threatening illnesses want to talk about their condition. Taking children's signals seriously requires good cooperation between parents and nurses in particular. Not only are nurses primarily responsible for most of children's care, but their daily contact with young patients also often means that they are in the best position to understand certain questions or interpret a state of suppressed despair.

A fundamental principle of dealing with hospitalised children is to minimise special treatment and sentimental expressions of sympathy in handling the issue of illness. Children are often grateful if their parents, instead of talking about the illness, distract them by reading aloud and generally behave as normally as possible.

15.2 Disabilities and chronic illnesses

Opportunities for development

The experiential realm of children who are born blind or lose their eyesight through accidents is limited by the absence of the dimension of light and colour; only through their sense of touch can they develop mental images of the objects around them. Their other senses compensate for the absence of sight by becoming stronger and more sensitive to details. Hence hearing and touch become much keener and more precise in visually impaired children than in sighted individuals, making these children more receptive to the inner character of a person's tone of voice or any other auditory expression. Moods and subtle soul gestures are often literally 'overlooked' by people who can see; blind people, however, are often much more attuned to them.

Raising children who are deaf has particular challenges, especially in relation to developing their ability to express thoughts and emotions. Sign language has helped a lot, but some parents can struggle to draw children out of their soul world. A deaf child may feel that a deep and emotional type of perception is inaccessible to them.

How do children experience the world when they are confined to a wheelchair, limp, cannot run, or are missing limbs? We often find that children with impaired mobility have above-average emotional energy, as if all the pent-up will that cannot be transformed into bodily activity becomes available in their capacity for emotion. This phenomenon is also evident in children with cleft palates or harelips. Because of some genetic or other predisposition, certain forces needed for shaping the skeleton have not been channelled into shaping the body and instead remain available for soul activity. As a result, raising such children is not always easy. They often seem to be 'bursting at the seams' and easily get carried away because they have not yet learned to manage their excess of emotional forces.

Other children have to cope with congenital or acquired damage to internal organs. Children who suffer from diabetes from a young age learn to gauge their food and physical activity much more consciously and take much more responsibility for themselves at an early age. By dealing with insulin injections and blood sugar testing and learning to assess their metabolic status, their families learn to substitute conscious thought and action for the cellular function (insulin production) that was destroyed by an autoimmune disorder in their pancreas.

Or, for example, an 11-year-old girl is taken to the doctor because she has stopped growing and is always pale and tired. The doctor discovers that her kidneys are only barely functioning and will eventually shut down due to a congenital, progressive condition. What

is life like on dialysis? What is the significance of having an organ transplant? What is the meaning of this type of illness?

How do we deal with children with heart defects, juvenile diabetes, rheumatic disease, asthma, psoriasis or cancer? The main premise of this book – that child development and overcoming disease are related processes – can be helpful in coming to grips with these serious questions. Each illness conceals a specific task, a unique opportunity for development, learning and mastery. Learning to recognise this opportunity is the first step in addressing the task. The task, however, cannot be generalised; each individual discovers and experiences it differently. For example, we cannot assume that all blind people have the same underlying challenges to face. At this point, therefore, we would like to present a few thoughts that can provide helpful direction in individual cases.

Living a 'normal' life

When faced with a child's illness or a disability, we must first learn to deal with our own fear, anxiety and worry, at least to a certain extent. In the process, it may be helpful to ask ourselves what aspects of the world a child with a disability or chronic illness experiences differently, and perhaps uniquely, as a result of their limitations: 'How can I help my child learn something essential from the experience of disability?' If we manage to achieve this attitude, the insights that result are much more likely to be useful in coping with the child's situation.

An important point to consider is that preschool children experience their disability only to the extent that adults allow them to do so. They often become aware of it only through their parents' fear, inappropriate overprotection or when adults discuss their illness in their presence or pamper them with expressions of regret and sympathy. But children with disabilities, if simply given the necessary care with a no-nonsense and matter-of-fact attitude and otherwise treated just like their siblings, will experience themselves as 'normal'. They will identify with their condition and find ways to cope with it without sensing that they are 'different'. This attitude lays the foundation for an inner confidence that they will most certainly need at some point.

When children are teased for the first time, for example, because they limp or are cross-eyed, or if they notice that people choose not to sit next to them on the bus because they think eczema is contagious, it is especially important for parents to convey to children that such experiences are quite natural and nothing to worry about. 2- to 4-year-olds can be distracted with a story or an activity or something to look at. To an older child, we can say, 'That boy doesn't know you at all. He wouldn't behave like that if he knew what you're really like.' Or, 'There's always something about everybody that other people can make fun of. Let's not get upset about it.'

We can also tell older children stories such as *The Ugly Duckling* or *Bearskin*, which describe how learning to bear the burden of looking different from other people transforms into something exceptionally beautiful and valuable. We can also tell them how an oyster copes with the pain of a foreign object getting inside its shell: it coats the object with mother-of-pearl to make it harmless, and the end product is a gleaming, pinkish-white pearl!

Depending on their situation and maturity, children of school age may be able to discuss their disability or chronic illness openly with their parents. In our daily life together, we can at least make it clear to them, in the case of diabetics, for example, that we value their ability, gained through dealing with illness, to take responsibility for their own bodies.

At an early age, chronically ill children gain the self-confidence to lobby for their disabilities in society and to seek out people who will help them with their unique tasks in life. In these conversations, the issue of fairness is bound to come up. For example, why do other children have it easier? But then, why does one person enjoy a life of ease and luxury while another lives in dire poverty? Why do external or personal circumstances allow one person to travel to distant countries and have great learning experiences while another is denied a similar opportunity? Such questions are challenging not only for those with disabilities or illnesses but also for healthy people. None of us is exempt from the need to come to grips with personal destiny. Chapter 7 on the purpose of childhood illnesses contains more discussion on this issue (see page 127).

15.3 Finding purpose in illness and disability

During their children's visits to the doctor, parents sometimes ask questions that are part of a larger context, including those about the meaning or purpose of specific diseases.

Pain and development

The experience of pain and suffering can enrich human lives and lead to new developmental possibilities. This is not true of animals. Because the behaviour of mature animals is almost perfectly adapted to their circumstances, undergoing illness or suffering pain cannot make a lion more perfectly lion-like or a dog more dog-like. In contrast, the pain and suffering we encounter on life's journey can alert human beings to new opportunities for development, and we can continue to become 'more human' as long as we live.

Although the doctor's task is to do everything possible to relieve suffering and bring about healing, enduring painful experiences is an essential part of human existence, as is death.

Freedom and necessity

We all feel 'unfree' when we have to learn something. How much lack of freedom, for instance, is involved in preparing for an exam? Did anyone ever learn to do arithmetic without obeying mathematical laws? Once we have passed the exam or learned arithmetic, however, our freedom increases because our ability has grown. The same is true with any necessity of destiny: it simply defines the circumstances needed for acquiring a specific ability.

From this perspective, every illness also represents a necessity, a condition under which we can acquire an ability that we will later be able to use freely. The first rule of treating illness, therefore, is to do everything possible so that the patient can reap the benefits of the experience and (if at all possible) be led towards healing. After all, the only possible meaning and purpose of illness is to become healthy again in body, soul and spirit, with refreshed consciousness and enhanced capabilities. Our task is to support this process.

Destiny and reincarnation

How can we understand and affirm a person's destiny, their purpose in life, when it's impossible for them to have a job, a family or their own independence? If the answer to these questions was, 'Serious disabilities have no meaning or purpose. These children cannot develop in any way,' everything that can be said about the human spirit and its destiny would be called into question. At this point, we would like to pose a different question, namely, 'What perspectives lead us on from here?'

Rudolf Steiner asserted that the experience of illness and pain is significant for spiritual development. He saw illness as a physical projection of spiritual experience or, 'the physical imagination (image) of spiritual life'.[13]

Nothing that a human individual undergoes and experiences is ever lost; it forms part of their further development. Could it be that the unfree experience of suffering through illness in one earthly life manifests in a future life as an inborn soul-spiritual talent?

Religion speaks of God's unfathomable will and of his grace, which compensates us in the hereafter for what we have been denied in this life. The question of our own continued existence after death, however, can never be satisfactorily answered by physical evidence. More decisive is our own experience: Does it lead us to see the possible truth in this idea? Do we experience that much in life remains obscure and incomprehensible if we reject the idea of reincarnation? Or, does the thought of repeated earthly lives help us understand and support destinies such as those of people with severe disabilities? If the answer is yes, we have a direct experience of the efficacy and thus also the reality of the concept of reincarnation. Here are two clarifying examples:

Imagine meeting a child who can neither speak nor walk. Lying in bed or sitting in a wheelchair, she is totally dependent on those around her. She spends an entire lifetime receiving their help; she emits sounds of comfort or discomfort, but she is incapable of 'doing' anything.

A 16-year-old boy enjoys working under supervision and works tirelessly. His speech is awkward, his expression is open. At his care home, he helps in the garden and does the same tasks every day in the house. He performs these simple tasks with a pleasure that contrasts starkly with the attitude of many 'normal' people, who approach their daily work as if they would rather be doing something completely different.

Approaching these destinies by asking what these people can learn in their present lives and what capacities they are developing for future earthly lives points us in a very productive direction. Teachers, special educators, doctors and therapists who take this approach enhance their options for supporting children and their parents.

We may realise, for example, that the girl in the first example is experiencing a lifetime of receiving, a whole life in which to learn that we must receive as well as give, that we owe all of our own possibilities to other people and to the world in which we live and act. After spending an entire life unable to do anything except receive and be dependent on her surroundings, in her next life she will certainly not make the mistake of believing that she does not need other people.

The young man who spends a lifetime working gladly and regularly is undergoing an especially intensive training of the will. Nothing strengthens the will more effectively than regular activity performed with complete sympathy. Just as our muscles need daily activity to grow strong, so too our will needs constant practice. In view of the absence of enthusiasm or strong intentions that we can observe in many people today, it is like a ray of hope to imagine the strength of purpose that can develop through such exceptional will training.

Teachers, therapists and doctors who work with such thoughts and questions, have a greater possibility of helping children with disabilities or chronic illnesses, as well as being able to support their parents. The concept of reincarnation is anything but an 'ideology of retribution'. Rather, it offers opportunities for us to further our own development and that of the world.

The educator Michael Bauer

once formulated this future-oriented aspect of the concept of reincarnation like this: 'The idea of reincarnation is a postulate of love. Those who truly want to help will not grow tired in a single earthly life.' This view of reincarnation emphasises not its fateful aspect, but the free will that allows us to take the situation that is given to us and make it meaningful for ourselves and for the world around us.

As part of this same line of thought, we must apply questions of destiny not only to illnesses and disabilities but also to talents and genius. We often accept our own gifts and abilities as matters of course. But do we know how we achieved them? Could it be that the things we are so proud of in ourselves or admire in others can be traced back to disabilities or illnesses in earlier lives?

As a rule, sick people grasp such issues more easily than healthy people do. Parents and doctors experience repeatedly that people affected by chronic illness or disability deal with these questions very differently from the sympathetic people around them. They often sense that their suffering belongs to them and is part of the current manifestation of their personality. At times this goes so far that they themselves comfort those who grieve for them. This 'victory' over illness is a sign of instinctive, subconscious understanding of the necessities of personal destiny.

On the other hand, it is only natural for people with chronic illnesses or disabilities to experience anger and denial and to refuse to accept their condition. This attitude is difficult to transform or overcome if people's education and life experience constantly confront them with the view that illness and suffering are meaningless coincidences in life and that everyone has a 'right to health'.

We see it as one of the essential tasks of education to foster an attitude that unites all of life's many different elements into a single meaningful field of experience, and approaches even the problematic elements from the perspective of what can be learned from them.

15.4 Ethical issues

Earlier in this chapter we shared our strong belief that there is no such thing as a meaningless illness or a life not worth living. Almost no question leads us so deeply into matters of destiny as the issue of good deeds. The Greek-derived word 'ethics' means a doctrine of good behaviour and good actions.

Here, too, scientific discussion, especially in the field of medicine, has faced increasing difficulties in recent decades.

As soon as our perspectives on human life expand to consider the human body, soul and spirit as extending beyond birth and death, ethical questions are transformed into questions of individual responsibility for one's own destiny and the destiny of others, leading to questions such as:

• What does terminating a pregnancy mean for the unborn child, the mother and the doctor who performs the abortion?

• What does brain death or donating or receiving an organ transplant mean for the human body, soul and spirit?

One's motive for action then takes centre stage. After all, motive is what determines the quality of an act. What are the real reasons for or against a particular immunisation, a specific therapy, or terminating a pregnancy? What personal, professional or health-related motives are at work?

Any system of ethics that takes the human soul and spirit seriously never asks about the act itself without also asking about the motives that lead to it and about the individual's relationship to its consequences. In addition to insight and understanding, profound fears, concerns, anger, love, trust and hope shape ethical reality and influence the quality of an action. The consequences of such actions, however, constitute the destiny of children and adults. For example, parents who have their child vaccinated against measles out of fear of encephalitis need to know that encephalitis can also be triggered by other infections.

The pre-eminent issue in this case is *how* to support children with our own best forces, *how* we develop confidence in their destiny and attempt to help them find their way into their body and into their own life. We surround our decision with thoughts and feelings that strengthen children's experience of existence and their constitutional state of health. Each decision, however, may have both positive and negative consequences. There is virtually no such thing as a 'perfect' decision.

For example, if my hope in having my child vaccinated against measles is to prevent possible damage, of course my motivation sounds good. On the other hand, by having her immunised I also deprive her of an opportunity to exert herself in coming to grips with this illness, an opportunity that would result in more permanent immunity and a better match between her body and her incarnating soul and spirit. In each decision, a great deal depends on how we live with its consequences. To what extent can we stand behind the positive consequences of our actions and counteract any negative consequences?

From this perspective, it is becoming increasingly impossible for ethics to take direction from existing values and norms. Normative ethics are in the process of being transformed into individual ethics. Regardless of the legalities that apply, each action must always be judged individually, and an individual must take responsibility for it.

The same is true of legislative regulation of organ transplants. Even when brain death is the legal criterion for organ removal, the donor, the receiver and the doctors performing the operation are linked in relationships of destiny that the participants should enter into deliberately and responsibly. This judgment must always be left to the individuals involved and potential donors and recipients must grapple with the issues in advance, so their decisions are made as freely and responsibly as possible.

Prenatal diagnosis

Today we are aware of a number of hereditary illnesses and congenital malformations that can be predicted with the help of prenatal diagnosis. In addition to ultrasound diagnosis of congenital malformations, diagnostic options in the first three months now include a computer-generated risk analysis based on a combination of specific blood tests in the mother and nuchal translucency measurement in the unborn child.

Other options include placental puncture and amniocentesis (which can damage a healthy baby or cause miscarriage in 1% of cases), which supply genetic material for diagnosing chromosomal abnormalities such as those indicated in Down's syndrome and Prader-Willi syndrome, and diseases such as cystic fibrosis that are associated with specific genes.

The purpose of prenatal diagnosis is usually not to treat the illness it reveals, which is generally impossible, but to permit timely termination of the pregnancy. Laws on termination of pregnancy vary in different countries (or states). It has never been proved that caring for children with disabilities or chronic illnesses severely compromises their parents' mental health. Nonetheless, this medical indication is invoked on a daily basis for aborting babies who would be born with illnesses and disabilities. The destinies concealed by this statistic do not employ lobbyists and therefore remain nameless and unknown. Ethical questions are always also questions of very individual destinies that have both a past and consequences for the present and future.

If *in utero* diagnostics are recommended to prevent malformed, congenitally ill or otherwise seriously disabled children from being born, the underlying assumption is that such lives are not worthy of human beings. On the other hand, if we believe that human beings exist before birth and that even a life of severe disability has meaning and purpose, the question acquires another dimension and the decision becomes more difficult to make.

From the perspective of individual destiny, the often despairing question: 'Why me? Why is my child suffering?' leads to other questions: 'Why do you need me in particular?' 'What connects me to you?' 'What can I do to further your destiny?' 'What do my own experiences and insights owe to you and your suffering?'

Of course no one actively wishes for illness or for a chronically ill child. But the modern medical achievements of prenatal diagnosis make it appear that we have a choice. If we accept that human beings exist before birth and after death (see page 290), this freedom of choice, however, is illusory, because the baby, whether healthy, disabled or ill, is already there. If we don't want a baby the way he is and send him back into prenatal life, what suffering are we inflicting by depriving him of the possibility of incarnating?

Thoughts of this sort are not simply questions for parents and experts; they affect us all. Even if it is more comfortable to leave decisions for and against *in utero* diagnostics, genetic manipulation or experimental cloning to experts, religious leaders or the government, every adult citizen needs to work on these questions. This is the only way to develop a sense of responsibility based on personal insight, which is the foundation of what Steiner called 'ethical individualism'.

16. External Treatments for Home Nursing

By Petra Lange

More so than is the case with adults, children's illness or health can be influenced via all of their senses. We can take wonderful healing advantage of this receptivity by using external applications: In combination with the right degree of warmth, substances work through the skin deep into all the organs and their functions. For example, free breathing can be restored, mucus dissolved, fever regulated and pain eased, while at the same time we are creating soothing sensory experiences instead of drug-induced side effects.

16.1 Compresses and poultices

Every compress or poultice consists of at least two cloths: an inner cloth of silk, linen or cotton, and a larger cloth for the outer covering. Wool is best for the outer cloth. For children who are sensitive to wool, use a thin cotton or silk cloth inside the woollen outer layer so it doesn't scratch.

Compress cloths should be as wrinkle-free as possible. Outer layers made of wool felt and knit scarves are especially easy to handle.

Secure the wrappings tightly so the compress doesn't shift when the child moves.

Here are some recommendations on suitable cloth to use:
- *Silk:* ideally raw silk (a medium-weight, grainy, linen-like silk made from short waste fibres).
- *Linen:* a dishtowel, for example.
- *Cotton:* gauze nappies, brushed cotton or flannel, handkerchiefs.
- *Wool:* scarves of soft virgin wool (you can knit one from merino wool in k1, p1 ribbing); felted, woven virgin wool fabrics; or combed, unspun fleece wool.

Choosing the inner cloth

- *Damp compresses:* fairly thick linen, brushed cotton or flannel, thick gauze nappies, or a double layer of raw silk.
- *Oil and ointment compresses:* thinner raw silk, thin gauze nappies, or handkerchiefs.
- *Quark poultices: a* highly absorbent middle layer, such as brushed cotton or flannel or fleece wool is absolutely necessary.
- **Caution:** quark (fermented skimmed milk) causes matting of woollen fabrics.

16.2 Ear problems

Chamomile bag

- **For mild earache**
- **For aftercare of inner ear infections**
- Place a handful of dried chamomile flowers in the centre of a thin cloth and secure the cloth with thread to make a small bag. Knead the bag briefly to break the flower heads into smaller pieces so the bag will conform to the shape of the ear.
- Heat the bag between 2 plates placed like a lid on top of a pot of boiling water. This method of heating preserves the etheric oils, and stops the bag from getting wet.
- When the bag is warmed through, place it on the child's ear, cover it with cotton or a piece of fleece wool and secure it with a wool scarf or cap.
- *Duration:* at least half an hour, or overnight.
- *For aftercare:* can be repeated for 2 weeks.
- Chamomile flowers have a pleasant smell and are very popular with children. The bag can be reused 4 or 5 times before the flowers lose their scent.

Onion bag

- **For severe earache**
- Onion bags reliably relieve pain and inhibit inflammation.
- Finely chop a medium-sized onion and wrap it in a thin cloth to make a roll as thick as your finger. (*Tip:* If you pack the onion into a gauze tube bandage and knot the ends, the onion cubes will not fall out even if the child tosses and turns.)
- The roll should be at body temperature; apply it to the child's ear and the area behind the ear.
- Cover it with cotton or fleece wool to absorb excess onion juice and fasten it securely in place with a wool scarf, a bandana or a thin wool cap.
- *Duration:* half an hour or longer, depending on skin sensitivity. May be applied several times a day. 30-minute treatments

repeated at intervals of 1–2 hours throughout the day are especially effective.

Alternative onion treatment

- Use a garlic press to squeeze 5–10 drops of juice out of a few onion cubes onto a small wad of cotton. Warm the wad in your hand and carefully insert it into the outer ear. Leave it in place for a minimum of 1 hour or overnight.

16.3 Throat poultices

Eucalyptus

- **For lymph node inflammation**

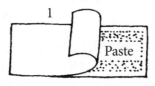

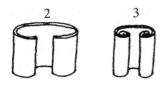

- Spread eucalyptus paste (*Eucalyptus comp.*) on a raw silk or cotton cloth long enough to cover the throat but somewhat shorter than the circumference of the child's neck (the cloth should leave 2 finger-widths exposed on either side of the neck vertebrae).

- Cover the paste with another cloth of the same size (1).
- Roll the poultice up from both ends towards the middle (2, 3) and heat it between 2 plates as described for the chamomile bag (see page 294).
- Test the temperature of the poultice on the inside of your lower arm.
- Press the poultice, still rolled up, briefly against your child's throat several times to make sure the temperature is comfortable, then unroll it in both directions, beginning at the larynx, and wrap it around your child's throat as smoothly as possible. Secure it with a woollen cloth, which will also prevent the poultice from cooling too quickly.
- *Duration:* overnight.

Onion ointment

- **For persistent cough**
- Warm about 100 g (4 oz) of goose fat, mix in a crushed or grated onion and allow it all to cool.
- Apply a layer of ointment as thick as a knife blade to a raw silk or cotton cloth that is long enough to cover the throat but leave the neck vertebrae exposed.
- Apply the ointment side of the cloth directly to the skin and secure it firmly with a layer of woollen cloth.

- The cloth can be reused several times.
- Each day, add enough ointment to make the surface of the cloth greasy.
- *Duration:* 1–2 hours unless skin irritation occurs sooner.

Archangelica comp. ointment

- **For lymph node inflammation or swollen glands**
- Instructions as above for Onion ointment.
- *Duration:* all day or overnight unless skin irritation develops.

Cool lemon juice

- **For acute sore throat with high fever**
- Place half of an unwaxed (preferably organic) lemon in a small bowl, cover it with water, make a few cuts in it and press the juice out with the bottom of a glass. (If only sprayed lemons are available, use a citrus juicer and dilute the juice with water.)
- Cut or fold a thin raw silk or cotton cloth so that it is long enough to cover the throat but leave the neck vertebrae exposed.
- Roll the cloth up from both ends towards the middle and saturate it with the lemon water.
- Wring it out and unroll it as smoothly as possible around

your child's throat, beginning at the larynx. Secure it firmly with a wool scarf.
- *Duration:* 1 hour or longer, depending on skin sensitivity.

Hot lemon juice

- **For milder sore throat or hoarseness**

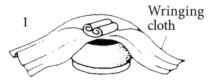

Wringing cloth

1

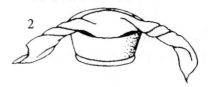

2

- Place half of an unwaxed (preferably organic) lemon in a small bowl, cover it with very hot water, make a few cuts in it and hold it in place with a fork while you press the juice out using the bottom of a drinking glass. (If you must use a sprayed lemon, extract the juice with a citrus juicer and dilute it with hot water.)
- Cut or fold a raw silk or cotton cloth (not too thin) to the right size to cover the throat but leave the neck vertebrae exposed.
- Roll the cloth up from both ends towards the middle, wrap it in a longer piece of cloth (1) and dip

both cloths into the hot lemon water, leaving the ends of the longer cloth dry (2).

- Pick up the ends of the longer cloth, drape it around a tap and twist the ends together to wring it out thoroughly. The drier the hot compress, the more comfortable it will be on the skin.
- Remove the compress from the wringing cloth.
- Test the temperature before unrolling it onto your child's throat, beginning at the larynx.
- The compress should be as wrinkle-free as possible.
- Secure it firmly with a wool scarf.
- *Duration:* at least 5–10 minutes.

Lemon slices
- **For tonsillitis**

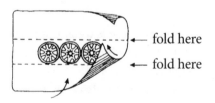

- This compress is more effective than those made with lemon juice, but also more irritating to the skin.
- Cut an unwaxed (preferably organic) lemon into thin slices.
- Wrap it in a cloth (not too thick) and squeeze it hard to extract some of the juice.

- Apply the poultice and secure it with a wool scarf.
- As with other throat applications, the neck vertebrae should not be covered.
- *Duration:* 20–60 minutes (maximum), depending on skin sensitivity. Remove the poultice if it begins to itch.

Quark
- **For tonsillitis with swelling**

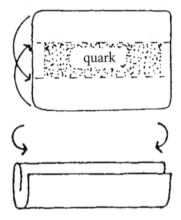

- A quark poultice is very soothing for when your child has a sore, swollen throat, a bad taste in their mouth and a high fever.
- **Do not use for children with eczema or dairy produce allergy.**
- Apply the quark (fermented skimmed milk) to a raw silk or cotton cloth.
- Use a thinner or thicker layer of quark depending on the patient's constitution. For a child

who tends to feel cold, use a thinner layer; otherwise, use a layer approximately 5 mm (¼ in) thick.

- Fold the cloth into a packet. There should be only one layer of cloth on the side that will be applied to the skin.

- Warm the poultice to room temperature between 2 hot-water bottles (not too hot to avoid making the quark too runny) until the outside of the poultice is hand-warm.

- Wrap it around the child's throat, leaving the neck vertebrae exposed.

- Secure it with a cotton or linen cloth, followed by an insulating layer of fleece wool wrapped in another cloth. Add another layer of wool cloth for the final covering.

- *Duration:* up to 8 hours, until the quark layer dries out. After removing the poultice, keep the patient's throat covered for a while with a scarf or turtleneck.

16.4 Chest poultices, compresses and rubs

Poultice with mustard

- **For obstructive bronchitis, asthma and pneumonia**
- **Use only as directed by a doctor!**

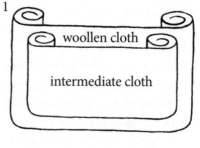

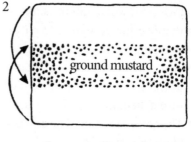

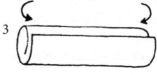

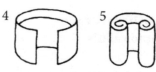

- This treatment is usually applied once a day in the evening to help children fall asleep.

- **A mustard poultice is a very powerful treatment that must be applied very carefully. Never use oil of mustard.**

- Mustard freshly ground before use is most effective. Mustard seed contains oil and is sensitive to heat. Do not grind it in a grain mill and avoid overheating it if you use an electric coffee grinder.

- Prepare the poultice in a warm room.
- Lay a wool cloth and an intermediate layer on the bed where the child's back will be (1).
- Spread a layer of ground mustard seed on a thin cloth that fits the area to be treated. The layer should be as thick as the blade of a knife (2).
- Fold and roll the cloth as illustrated here in Figures 2 and 3. The ground mustard should not escape from the cloth.
- The poultice can be applied to the shoulder blades, chest or both, but it is most effective if it wraps all the way around the ribcage (4).
- Moisten the poultice thoroughly with warm water (no hotter than 38°C/100°F) immediately before applying. If you're using a small cloth moisten with a spray. If you're using a large cloth, roll it up from both ends (5), submerge it briefly in lukewarm water, and carefully press our excess water with your hand. Do not wring.
- Protect the patient's nipples and armpits with petroleum jelly and cotton wool.
- Your child should sit up in bed as the poultice is unrolled smoothly onto the skin in both directions, beginning at the spine.
- Next, ask your child to lie down on the previously prepared cloths and secure them firmly around the upper body.
- Add a sweater over the top, as well as dressing your child warmly all over or wrapping in a blanket.
- Your child should to lie by an open window while the poultice does its work.
- A warm, burning sensation soon develops over the ribcage, which can cause young children to cry, but this is actually helpful for the lungs.
- *Duration:* it usually takes about 4 minutes to produce the desired level of skin reddening. If there is no reddening, increase the time by 2 minutes at a time, up to a maximum of 8 minutes.
- Return your child to a warm bed before removing the poultice.
- Rub a mild vegetable oil into the treated area, making sure that no traces of mustard remain on the skin.
- If the child's skin is still red the next day or show signs of pimples, substitute an oil compress and do not repeat the mustard treatment until the following day.
- If the skin does not redden, check whether the ground mustard is too old. Using overly hot water to moisten the poultice also reduces the effect.

- Make a new mustard poultice for each application.
- Once you have experienced the beneficial effects of this poultice, you will find it well worth the effort to make it and to help your child through the few minutes of burning warmth.

Compress with ginger

- **For obstructive bronchitis, persistent cough**
- Measure ¼ litre (1 US cup) of hot water.
- In a small bowl, mix 2 teaspoons of grated fresh ginger root or ground ginger thoroughly with 4 tablespoons of the water.
- Cover it and set aside to steep for 10 minutes.
- Meanwhile, prepare the compress cloths: a raw silk or cotton cloth large enough to completely cover the child's ribcage is rolled up from both ends towards the middle and wrapped in a larger cloth to make it easier to wring out (see page 296).
- Pour the rest of the water over the ginger, dip the cloths into the ginger-water mixture, keeping the ends of the outer cloth dry. Loop the cloth over a tap and twist hard to wring it out.
- Spread the outer woollen covering on the child's bed.
- Make sure the compress is not too hot before applying it.

- With the child sitting in bed, roll the compress out smoothly from the spine in both directions to cover the entire ribcage.
- Have the child lie down on the wool cloth and use it to secure the compress firmly in place.
- As with a mustard poultice, do not apply just before your child is going to sleep, as the loosened phlegm first needs to be coughed up. A lavender oil compress is more suitable for evenings (see page 301).
- *Duration:* 5 minutes for the first application. If no skin irritation occurs, increase the time by 3 minutes at each application, but do not exceed 20 minutes.
- The patient should be in a warm bed when you remove the compress. Rub the treated area gently with a mild vegetable oil.
- The ginger-water mixture should not be used more than once. Ground ginger may be available from a herbalist under the name *rhizoma zingiberis pulvis* or from a general store.

Compress with beeswax

- **For colds, coughs, bronchitis**
- This compress is a favourite with parents and children because it is simple to use. We recommend ready-to-use compresses, but if you prefer to make the compress yourself, make sure you use

beeswax with minimal contaminants.

- Dip a piece of thin raw silk or cotton cloth (about 20 x 15 cm / 8 x 6 in) 2 or 3 times in wax melted over a hot water bath. Allow each layer of wax to dry briefly before dipping again.
- Lay the compress on a cloth-covered layer of wool batting or the silk-and-wool sack provided in the ready-to-use compress kit and then heat it up with a hair dryer until it is flexible but not too hot.
- Now lay the compress on your child's skin, cover it with the wool batting or sack to hold the warmth in and secure everything with a wool scarf.
- *Duration* 30 minutes to 2 hours, up to twice a day, if your child's skin tolerates it.
- After use, the cloth can be stored wrapped in waxed paper and then sealed in a plastic bag to retain the scent. It can be reused as long as the wax smells pleasant and doesn't crumble.

Compress with etheric oils (10% lavender, 10% eucalyptus or dwarf-pine)

- **For bronchitis, obstructive bronchitis, croup, pneumonia or whooping cough**

- Chest compresses with etheric oils, especially lavender oil with its pleasant scent and calming effects, are great favourites with parents and children alike.
- For use on sensitive skin, dilute the etheric oil with an equal amount of vegetable oil (cold-pressed, if possible) or saturate the compress cloth with vegetable oil and sprinkle on a few drops of the 10% etheric oil, gradually increasing the amount if your child tolerates it.
- On aluminium foil, place a raw silk or cotton cloth, large enough to go completely round the ribcage.
- Add 5–10 ml (½–1 tablespoon) of oil.
- Roll up from both sides so that the foil wraps around the cloth, then warm between 2 hot-water bottles.
- Remove the cloth from the foil and quickly wrap it around the patient's ribcage, beginning at the back and secure it firmly with a wool scarf.
- Do not use plastic instead of foil, as the etheric oils may absorb some of the plastic.
- *Duration:* at least half an hour if applied during the day, but overnight is better.
- The oil-saturated cloth can be reused as long as it still smells good (2 weeks or longer). After

each use, store it in the used aluminium foil in a cool place. Freshen it up with a little new oil before each use.

Chest rub with etheric oils (10% lavender, 10% eucalyptus or dwarf-pine)

- **For bronchitis, obstructive bronchitis, croup, pneumonia or whooping cough (as an alternative to a chest compress)**
- A chest rub requires calm, concentrated movements with *warm* hands and *very small amounts* of oil.
- Rub the entire ribcage with the oil of your choice and wrap the child's upper body in a wool cloth when you have finished the rub.
- (In New Zealand, Eucalyptus comp. chest paste or Eucalytus/ Plantago comp. chest rub are available.)

Chest rubs with damp compresses

- **For bronchitis, obstructive bronchitis, croup, pneumonia or whooping cough**
- After a chest rub, the effect can be enhanced by adding a damp compress.
- Use a piece of raw silk or cotton cloth as wide as the child's chest.

- Roll the cloth up from both sides towards the middle, place it inside a larger cloth (see page 298).
- Pour hot water over it and then wring it out (grasp the larger cloth by the ends, sling it around a tap and twist firmly).
- Remove the compress from the outer cloth, place it on the treated skin and secure it firmly with a woollen cloth.
- *Duration:* after half an hour, loosen the woollen wrappings just enough to remove the compress. Leave the wool cloth in place while the patient rests for an hour, or even overnight.

Compress with horsetail (equisetum) tea

- **For bronchitis with a great deal of phlegm but no high fever**
- To make the tea, pour ½ litre (2 US cups) of water over a handful of dried horsetail (equisetum) herb, bring it to a boil and simmer for 10 minutes. Remove from heat and allow the tea to steep, covered, for 5 minutes longer while you get the compress cloths ready.
- *Alternative method, for stronger tea:* soak a handful of dried horsetail herb in ½ litre (2 US cups) of water for 10 hours, boil it for 5 minutes and let it steep covered for 5 minutes longer.

- Cut or fold a raw silk or cotton cloth (not too thin) to the right size to completely cover the ribcage.
- Roll the cloth up from both ends towards the middle, wrap it in a longer piece of cloth to aid wringing it out.
- Pour the tea through a strainer onto the cloth.
- Spread the outer woollen cloth on the child's bed.
- With the child sitting up in bed, unroll the compress smoothly onto their back in both directions, ending in front.
- Have the child lie down on top of the wool cloth and use it to secure the compress in place.
- *Duration:* after half an hour, loosen the wool wrapping slightly and quickly remove the compress. Leave the wool fabric in place while the patient rests for an hour (or overnight).
- If the skin is irritated by the wool, remove the woollen wrapper and put it back on again over a pyjama top. Move quickly to avoid losing heat.

Poultice with quark

- **For pneumonia, pleurisy and bronchitis with a great deal of phlegm**
- **Do not use for children with eczema or dairy produce allergy.**
- The size of the cloth used

depends on whether you wish to apply the poultice all the way around the ribcage or only to the patient's chest.

- Spread the quark (fermented skimmed milk) on a raw silk or cotton cloth (see page 297). The layer of quark should be about as thick as your little finger.
- Warm the quark poultice to skin temperature on a hot-water bottle (take care not to make it too hot or the quark will become too runny).
- To apply a poultice that wraps all the way around the torso, spread the outer woollen cloth and an absorbent intermediate layer on the child's bed, with the poultice on top. With the child lying on their back on the entire package, wrap both sides of the poultice around to the front, secure it firmly with the absorbent layer and cover it with the outer cloth.
- *Tip:* a layer of fleece wool wrapped in a cotton cloth makes a very warm and absorbent intermediate layer for a quark poultice, and a thinner cloth or even an undershirt can then be used for the outermost layer. Using fleece wool also avoids ruining a woollen cloth, which mats when in contact with the liquid from quark.
- *Duration:* leave the poultice in place until the layer of quark

dries out. How long this takes depends on the thickness of the quark layer and also varies from patient to patient (anywhere from 3–8 hours).

Heart compress with Aurum/Lavandula comp. cream

- **For nervous, anxious children who have trouble sleeping or falling asleep**
- Warm a small piece of silk or cotton cloth and spread the ointment on it in a thin layer. Apply the compress to the child's heart area at bedtime.
- As a rule, wearing an undershirt over the compress is enough to hold it in place.
- If extra warmth is needed, a woollen cloth can be wrapped around the ribcage over the compress.
- *Duration:* overnight.

16.5 Abdominal compresses

- **For certain types of abdominal pain and vomiting**
- **Appendicitis should be ruled out first.**
- Abdominal compresses are also a wonderful aid to falling asleep and can help insomnia.

Yarrow

- To make the tea, pour approximately ½ litre (2 US cups) of hot water over a handful of yarrow. Cover it and allow to steep for at least 10 minutes.
- Meanwhile, fold a cloth to the desired size and wrap it in a larger cloth to make it easier to wring out (see page 296).
- Pour the tea through a strainer onto the cloths.
- Wring out the cloths.
- Remove the compress from the outer cloth. It should be applied as hot as your child can tolerate.
- Secure it with a strip of cotton or linen long enough to wrap all the way around the body and add a woollen cloth as the outer covering. These cloths should be much wider than the compress so that no cool spots develop along the edges.
- Place 2 hot-water bottles (not bulging full) on top of the compress on either side of the stomach and pull the child's pyjama bottoms up over it to secure it.
- *Duration:* 30–60 minutes, then remove the compress from under the woollen cloth. The woollen cloth can remain in place while the patient rests for an hour (or overnight).

Chamomile

- Prepare in the same way as the yarrow compress. Use a handful of chamomile tea to ½ litre (2 US cups) of hot water.

Oxalis essence

- Prepare in the same way as the yarrow compress. Use 1 tablespoon of oxalis essence to approximately ¼ litre (1 US cup) of hot water.

Caraway or lemon-balm oil

- Prepare and apply like a chest compress with etheric oils (see page 301).

Copper ointment (0.4%) compress

- Apply copper ointment in a thin, very even layer to a piece of raw silk or cotton cloth. Don't spread it all the way to the edges.
- Secure the cloth to the area to be treated with a wool scarf tied around the child's body.
- *Duration:* **as prescribed by your doctor.**
- Following treatment, clean the skin with warm water and dry thoroughly.
- Like all metal ointments, copper produces stains that are hard to remove.
- The compress can be reused several times. Apply more ointment as needed (2 or 3 times a week).

Dry abdominal compress

- Place a dry, well-warmed cloth on the patient's abdomen and secure it firmly with a strip of wool cloth.

Liver compress with yarrow

- Prepare in the same way as the yarrow compress.
- Apply the compress to the skin over the liver (on the right side, from the navel around to the back).

16.6 Kidney and bladder treatments

Kidney compress with copper ointment

- **For asthma**
- **As directed by a doctor**
- Apply copper ointment in a thin, very even layer to a piece of raw silk or cotton cloth. Don't spread it all the way to the edges.
- Secure the cloth to the kidney area and secure it firmly with a wool scarf tied around the child's body.
- *Duration:* **as prescribed by your doctor.**
- Following treatment, clean the skin with warm water and dry thoroughly.
- Like all metal ointments, copper produces stains that are hard to remove.

- The compress can be reused several times. Apply more ointment as needed (2 or 3 times a week).
- Your doctor may also prescribe silver (Argentum) ointment to alternate with the copper ointment.

Bladder rub with 10% eucalyptus oil and moist compress

- **For early treatment of urinary tract infections**
- With a warm hand and using slow, careful movements, rub the bladder area with a very small amount of 10% eucalyptus oil.
- Roll up a palm-sized piece of raw silk or cotton cloth from both sides towards the middle. Then wrap it in a larger cloth to make it easier to wring out and pour hot water over it (see page 296).
- Wring it out. The drier the cloth, the hotter it can be applied to the skin.
- Remove the compress from the outer cloth, place it on the oiled area and cover it with a woollen cloth or fleece wool.
- Hold the compress in place with a pair of snug-fitting underpants.
- *Duration:* after half an hour, loosen the wool covering and remove the compress. Leave the wool in place while the patient rests for 1 hour (or overnight). Repeat this application several

times during the first and second days of the infection, then continue the treatment with eucalyptus oil compresses (see below).

Bladder compresses with 10% eucalyptus oil

- **For urinary tract infections**
- **Follow-up treatment after eucalyptus bladder rubs**
- Pour about 5 ml (½ tablespoon) of oil onto a palm-sized piece of raw silk or cotton cloth and warm as described for compress with etheric oils (see page 301).
- Place the oiled cloth over the bladder and cover it with a woollen cloth or a layer of fleece wool.
- Pull the child's underpants over it to hold it in place.
- *Duration:* Several hours once a day at least until symptoms are gone.
- The oil-saturated cloth can be reused as long as it still smells good (2 weeks or longer). After each use, store it in the used aluminum foil in a cool place. Freshen it up with a little new oil before each use.
- Your doctor may prescribe bladder compresses with silver ointment (Argentum metalicum prep. 0.4%) to alternate with eucalyptus compresses. Follow your doctor's instructions for preparation.

16.7 Treatment of the limbs and feet

Warm compresses with arnica essence

- **For rising fever if your child is restless, nauseous or has a headache or chills**
- For this treatment, you will need 4 pieces of raw silk or cotton cloth of the right size to wrap around your child's wrists and ankles.
- Roll each cloth up individually from both ends towards the middle and wrap 2 each in 2 larger cloths.
- Place both of the larger cloths in a bowl (see page 296) and pour over them a mixture of 1 tablespoon of arnica essence and approximately ¼ litre (1 US cup) of very hot water.
- Thoroughly wring out one set of cloths (see page 296).
- Apply the compresses to the inside of the wrists. First, take one of the inner cloths out of the large cloth, wrap it over one wrist and fasten it firmly with a woollen cloth. Then repeat for the second wrist.
- Similarly, apply a compress to each ankle, removing the compress cloths from their covering one at a time.
- *Duration:* repeat 3 times every 10 minutes, followed by a 1-hour pause. Remove as soon as the period of rising fever is over: that is, as soon as your child's limbs feel hot.

Tepid leg compresses

- **To reduce fever**

Tepid calf compresses are a reliable fever-reducing treatment. Since they usually need to be applied at night, here are a few tips for making the process easier:

- Prepare 4 cloths at once rather than 2, so that 2 new ones are already at hand when it is time to change the compresses.
- Remove each used cloth from its wrapping and apply a fresh one immediately, while the leg is still a bit damp.
- Linen works especially well for calf compresses. Unlike cotton, it is somewhat stiffer wet than dry and does not cause a constricting sensation as it dries.
- **If the patient has cold feet and/or cold legs, do not use these compresses even if their fever is high!**
- First, lay a thick cotton cloth such as a bath towel over the bed to protect the mattress. Pour 2 to 3 litres/quarts of water into a bowl. The water should be only very slightly cooler than the patient's measured body temperature.
- Adding lemon to the water

intensifies the effect of the compress. Slice half of an unsprayed (preferably organic) lemon into the water and squeeze hard to extract the juice. (If you must use a sprayed lemon, squeeze out the juice and measure 2 tablespoons into the water.) Alternatively, any fruit vinegar may be substituted for the lemon.

- Fold 2 cloths to a size that covers the child's leg from the ankle to just below the knee and wraps around the leg about 1 ½ times.
- Roll the cloths up from both ends and wet them thoroughly with the water.
- Before applying them, squeeze them out until they no longer drip.
- Wrap each leg from the ankle to the knee with one of the cloths, securing it with a large wool sock, a woollen scarf or a thick cotton cloth. Do not use foil, plastic or non-absorbent cloth.
- Keep the patient fully covered (including their legs) during the treatment; a light blanket or sheet is enough if their fever is high.
- *Duration:* after 5 or 10 minutes, the cloths will be warmed through and must be replaced with new ones. After 3 repetitions, wait for half an hour before continuing.

- **Discontinue treatment if the patient's feet get cold.**

Mustard footbath

- **For enlarged tonsils, inflammation of the nose, sinuses or throat**
- **Migraine**
- Tie 1 or 2 handfuls of freshly ground mustard seed into a thin cloth and place with the knot down into a bucket of water warmed to 37–39°C/98.5–102°F.
- *Duration:* the patient's feet should stay in the bath for up to 10 minutes. Wrap a bath towel around the container and over the patient's knees so the water does not cool down too fast. Do not have more than 1 footbath per day.
- Do not allow the bath mixture to come into contact with any mucous membranes. Wash your hands carefully after preparing the bath and rinse the patient's legs thoroughly when the footbath is over.
- This footbath produces significant skin reddening, although it may appear only after several applications.
- Conclude the treatment by rubbing the patient's legs with a mild plant-based body oil.

Ginger-salt footbath

- **For enlarged tonsils, inflammation of the nose, sinuses or throat**

- **Migraine**
- A ginger-salt footbath is often more readily tolerated by sensitive skin than a footbath with powdered mustard.
- Briefly boil 2 tablespoons of ground ginger in about ½ litre (quart) of water. If this amount is well tolerated, it can be increased to 4 tablespoons of ground ginger. Alternatively, use juice pressed from fresh ginger.
- Prepare a nice warm footbath and add the ginger mixture (or juice).
- *Duration:* about 10 minutes. Stop sooner if there is any burning sensation.
- Afterwards, rinse your child's feet with lukewarm water and apply sage oil (10% Oleum salviae) or olive oil.

Mustard poultices on the soles of the feet

- **An alternative to footbaths for very young or very restless children**
- For each poultice, tie 1 or 2 tablespoons of ground mustard in the centre of a thin but densely woven handkerchief. Thoroughly moisten these little bags in lukewarm water and then squeeze them out.
- Apply 1 bag to the sole of each foot, holding them in place with socks or larger cloths.
- *Duration:* until the skin reddens

(3–15 minutes; it varies from person to person).
- **Remove the poultice when a burning sensation develops.**
- After removing the poultices, rub the patient's feet with a good quality vegetable oil.
- Warm wool socks intensify the effect.

16.8 Cool compresses

- For these compresses, dilute 1 tablespoon of essence with 9 tablespoons of water.
- Saturate a fairly thick cloth (a double layer of raw silk or brushed cotton or flannel) with the liquid.
- Squeeze out the cloth until it no longer drips and apply it as smoothly as possible to the area to be treated.
- Fasten the compress with a woollen cloth or a thick cotton cloth.
- Use a spoon or a small jug to add more of the diluted essence to the compress as it dries.

Arnica essence

- **For bruises, sprains and strains**
- *Duration:* change the compress at least once a day.
- **Do not apply arnica compresses to broken skin, and do not use them if the patient is allergic to arnica.**

Calendula essence

- **For scrapes and oozing wounds**
- This compress is also a painless way to remove bandages that have stuck to wounds.
- *Duration:* change every hour, using freshly ironed inner cloths to help prevent infection. After several hours, let the wound air-dry.

Combudoron essence

- **For burns, insect bites or sunburn**
- **Caution is advised in using Combudoron on patients with known allergies to arnica.**
- This compress is good for relieving pain on the way to the doctor. It also removes bandages that have stuck to wounds.
- Use a freshly ironed inner cloth.
- *Duration:* change at least once a day.

Quark poultice

- **For milk retention, mastitis (only as directed by doctor or midwife)**
- **For sunburn, bruises, sprains and strains**
- **Do not use for children with dairy produce allergy.**
- Apply a thin layer (knife-blade thick) of skimmed milk quark to a thin raw silk or cotton cloth, as described for throat poultice with quark (see page 297).

- The size of the poultice cloth depends on the size of the area to be treated.
- In the case of a nursing mother with mastitis or milk retention, warm the poultice to skin temperature on a hot-water bottle (ensure it does not get too hot or the quark will curdle). Leave the mother's nipple exposed when you apply the poultice.
- *Duration:* remove the poultice approximately 20 minutes before nursing. Rubbing the breast gently with oil will warm it and stimulate milk flow.

16.9 Warm compresses

Compress with 10% calendula oil

- **For mumps**
- Warm a palm-sized piece of raw silk or cotton cloth on the radiator.
- Pour approximately 5 ml of calendula oil into a small, clean bottle and warm it in a hot water bath.
- Drip the oil onto the cloth until it is completely saturated. You can also saturate the cloth with unwarmed oil and heat the compress between 2 plates.
- The compress should be as warm as the patient can tolerate.
- Apply it to the swollen area,

secure it with a bandana and cover it with a woollen scarf.

- Fleece wool is especially good for this type of compress; use a layer under the bandana.
- *Duration:* several times a day for half an hour, or overnight.
- The oil-saturated cloth may be reused as long as it smells good (approximately 2 weeks). After each use, store it in a clean glass jar in a cool, dark place. Freshen it up with a little additional oil before each application.

Compress with horsetail (equisetum) tea

- **For severely oozing eczema**
- To make the tea, cover a handful of dried horsetail (equisetum) herb with 1 litre (quart) of cold water, bring to the boil and simmer for 10 minutes. Cover the tea and allow it to steep for 5 minutes while you get the cloths ready.
- *Alternative method, for stronger tea:* Soak a handful of dried horsetail herb in 1 litre (quart) for 10 hours, boil it for 5 minutes and let it steep covered for 5 minutes longer.
- Use a raw silk or cotton cloth of a size to cover the affected area. Soak it in the tea (which should be at body temperature or slightly warmer), squeeze it out and apply it as smoothly as possible.

- In this case, a wool wrapping is often not possible. Secure the compress with a larger cotton cloth (or better still, with a layer of fleece wool wrapped in a cotton cloth so that the wool is not in direct contact with the skin).
- *Duration:* at least half an hour. If the compress is left on longer, it may be necessary to remoisten the inner cloth by carefully adding more tea with a spoon.

16.10 Washes and baths

Cool washes

- **To strengthen the immune system**
- **Do not apply cool washes if your child's skin is not thoroughly warm.**
- Washed body parts must be dried and covered immediately to prevent evaporative cooling.
- Have your child sit up and slip out of their pyjamas.
- Spread a large bath towel on their bed for them to lie on, and cover them warmly.
- In a basin, mix a teaspoon of rosemary concentrate with about 2 litres/quarts of cool water. The water should not be so cool that it feels unpleasant.
- Dip a wash mitt (not a washcloth) into the water and wring

it out until it no longer drips. Wash your child's face first; a few strokes from the forehead to the neck are sufficient. Then wipe from the neck down the back in several strokes.

- After gently drying your child's back, have them lie down and cover them well.
- Next, refresh the wash mitt. Uncover your child's left arm and wipe it with large strokes, moving from their fingertips to their shoulder. Dry the arm immediately and cover it again. Repeat with the right arm.
- Then wash the ribcage in a few strokes from the neck to the ribs.
- Cover your child carefully up to their neck and have them stick their left leg out from under the covers. Wipe the leg using large strokes, moving from their toes upwards.
- Repeat with the right leg to finish the treatment.
- *Duration:* the whole procedure should not take more than 5 minutes. When finished, have your child rest in bed, well covered for half an hour.

Tepid sponge bath
- **To reduce fever**
- **If the patient has cold feet and/ or cold legs, do not use these compresses even if their fever is high!**

- A sponge bath with cool water (see the instructions on page 311) is even more effective if you use water with lemon.
- Don't dry your child after washing them down; simply cover them well.
- In many cases, washing the calves is enough.

Sweat packs
- **For the start of a cold**
- May be preceded by a warm bath, adding hot water gradually to increase the temperature, with a few drops of lemon added to the water.
- Give your child hot linden-flower (lime-flower) tea to drink.
- Have them put on a bathrobe if it seems necessary for warmth.
- Cover them very warmly in bed (up to their ears).
- *Duration:* after ½–2 hours, when your child has perspired freely and perhaps slept a little, rub them down with a damp, cool washcloth and change their pyjamas.

Steam inhalation
- **For respiratory infections: colds (with chamomile tea); coughs (with thyme tea)**
- **Do not use etheric oils!**
- Steam inhalation clears the nasal passages and prevents infections.
- Place 2 chairs on a table and lay

cloths over them to make a tent or cave.

- Place a wide, stable pot in the centre to hold the hot tea.
- Wrap a towel around the pot so your child can't touch its hot sides.
- In a tent like this, an adult can comfortably inhale steam with a baby, or an older child can do it alone.
- *Duration:* 5–10 minutes, or up to 15 minutes for older children. Then stay in a warm room for 1 hour.
- After the steam treatment, you may apply calendula or mercurialis ointment to your child's face.

Baths with horsetail (equisetum) tea

- **For hives, eczema (especially itching forms), neurodermatitis and to stimulate skin metabolism**
- Baths with *equisetum (horsetail) essence* stimulate elimination via the kidneys and are good for eczema (including the itching forms) and poorly healing wounds.
- Soak 50 g (1¾ oz) of horsetail (equisetum) herb in 2–3 litres (quarts) of cold water for 10 hours.
- Then bring to a boil and simmer for 10 minutes.
- *Faster alternative:* pour 2 litres

(quarts) of cold water over 100 g (3½ oz) of horsetail herb, bring to a boil, simmer for 5 minutes and steep covered for 15 minutes.

- Strain the tea into the bath water. The water should be at 35–36°C (95–97°F).
- *Duration:* spend 5–10 minutes in the bath.
- For hives, rinsing with cool water after the bath often feels good.

Baths with herbal essences

- Use Wala or Weleda essences, which are made from fresh, biodynamically grown medicinal herbs.
- Add 1 tablespoon of essence to a full bath. The water should be at 35–36°C (95–97°F).
- *Duration:* spend 5–10 minutes in the bath.

Baths with sea salt

- **For adenoids and susceptibility to upper respiratory infections**
- **Do not use during feverish illnesses.**
- **Do not use soap or shampoo during these baths.**
- The water temperature should be 35°C/95°F.
- Do not rinse the saltwater off: simply dry your child quickly or, better still, wrap them

immediately in a big bathrobe and put them to bed.

- **A 1–2-hour rest after the bath is a necessary part of the treatment.**
- The amount of salt used depends on the child's age, and both the amount of salt and the duration of the bath are increased during the series of baths:
- For children 3–12 years old, begin with 3 kg (6¼ lb) sea salt in 200 litres of bath water (50 US gallons). Do not simply estimate the amount of water; measure it in a 10-litre (2 gallon) bucket or similar.
- Keeping the same proportions, you can use less salt for a smaller

child who can be bathed in a smaller tub. The child must be able to lie comfortably in the tub, however and be completely covered by the bath water.

- *Duration:* the first 4 baths should each last 10 minutes. For baths 5 through to 8, increase the amount of salt by ⅓ and the length of the bath to 15 minutes. Beginning with bath 9, increase the *original* amount of salt by ⅔ and the length of the bath to 20 minutes.
- Sea salt baths should be administered 2 or 3 times a week. A complete saltwater course includes 14 baths.

Knitting and Sewing Patterns

Baby's woollen pants/ soakers

Size given is for between 4 and 14 months. (They tend to grow with the child!) For a smaller size use thinner knitting needles.

Materials
- 70 g (2.5 oz) pure untreated wool, double knitting thickness
- One pair each of No. 8 (4 mm) (5 US) and No. 10 (3.25 mm) (3 US) knitting needles
- One set of No. 10 (3.25 mm) (3 US) knitting needles

Front
- Cast on 60 sts. on No. 10 needles.
- Work 16 rows K2, P2.
- Change to No. 8 needles and work 48 rows in garter (plain) stitch.
- Change back to No. 10 needles and knit 8 rows K2, P2.
- Next 16 rows: K together the first two and the last two sts. of every row keeping K2, P2 rib intact. 28 sts.
- Knit 5 more rows in K2, P2 and cast off.

Back
Work as front.

Assembly
- Sew up side seams from waist down to where the ribbing starts.
- Sew up seam between legs.
- With set of No. 10 needles, pick up the end sts. around each leg (about 48 sts.).
- Make a K2, P2 border of 6 rounds.
- Cast off loosely.

Vest / sleeveless sweater

Size given is for about 6 months to 1 year. (Larger size 4–6 years in parentheses.)

Materials
- 50 g (2 oz) (100 g, 4 oz) soft 4-ply wool or silk
- One pair No. 9 (3.75 mm) (4 US) knitting needles

Front
- Cast on 50 (60) sts. and work 10 (14) rows in K2, P2.
- Knit 40 (63) rows in st.st. (K1, P1)

- Work the next 18 (39) rows in K2, P2.
- Next row, to shape neck opening: work 12 (14) sts. in K2, P2, cast off 26 (32) sts., work 12 (14) sts. in K2, P2.
- Knit 6 (12) rows with the 12 (14) sts. on each side, keeping the K2, P2 ribbing intact.
- Cast off.

Back
Work as front.

Assembly
- Press carefully.
- Join shoulder seams and side seams leaving an opening for the arms.

Baby's bonnet
- Size given is for about birth to 2 months. (Larger size 6–12 months in parentheses.)

Materials
- 30 g (1 oz) of 4-ply wool or cotton or silk
- One pair No. 11 (3 mm) (2 US) knitting needles (Larger size: No. 8/4 mm/5 US needles)

Pattern
- Cast on 60 (80) sts. and work 7 (8) rows in K1, P1.
- Carry on knitting in st.st. (K1, P1) until work measures 10 cm (4 in) (12.5 cm, 5 in), ending on a right-side row.
- Start to decrease as follows: first row * sl. 1, K1, psso, K8 *. Repeat from * to * to end of row, 54 sts. (72 sts.).
- Next and every alt. row: purl
- Third row: * sl. 1, K1, psso, K7 *. Repeat from * to * to end of row.
- Fifth row: * sl. 1, K1, psso, K6 *. Repeat from * to * to end of row.
- Continue in this way until you have 6 (8) sts. left.

Assembly
- Cut the yarn and thread through left-over sts.
- Sew up the back seam from the back of the bonnet to the row at which decreasing started.
- Crochet two lengths of string for tying on the bonnet and sew one on to each front corner.

Key

alt.	alternate
k.	knit
p.	purl
psso.	pass slip stitch over
rep.	repeat
sl.	slip
st(s).	stitch(es)
st.st.	stocking stitch

Cotton suit for eczema sufferers

Front of suit
Seam at the front

Sleeve
Cut twice. Fold and
sew each sleeve.

Side-piece with slit for sleeve
Cut twice. To find length: measure from shoulder to heel and add length of foot. Keep measurements generous for comfort. Sew the two side pieces together down the front seam and inside legs.

Back of suit
Open at the back. Close with cotton ribbons or ties.

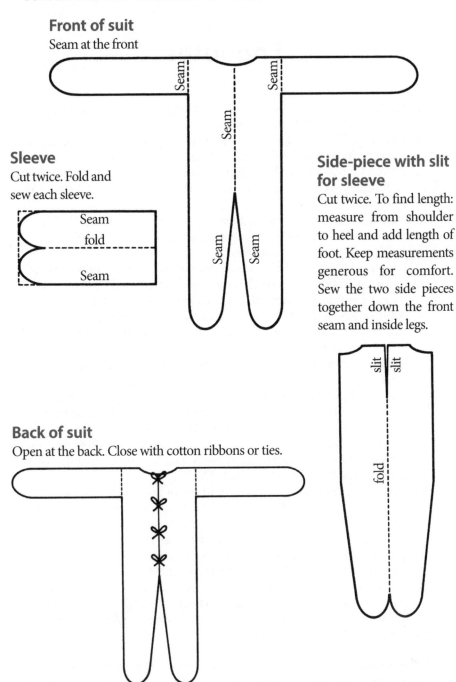

Endnotes

1. See Fingado, M., *Rhythmic Einreibung*, Floris Books, 2011 for instructions on rhythmical massage.
2. Flöistrup, H., Swartz J. et al. 'Allergic disease and sensitisation in Steiner school children', *Journal of Allergy and Clinical Immunology* 2006, 117: 59–66; and Von Alm, J., and J. Swartz, 'Atopy in children of families with an anthroposophical lifestyle', *Lancet* 1999, 353: 1485–88
3. Steiner, R. *Verses and Meditations*, Rudolf Steiner Press, UK 1972
4. See: www.childrenwithcancer.org.uk/childhood-cancer-info/childhood-cancer-facts-figures
5. Längler, A. Spix, C. et al. 'Anthroposophical medicine in paediatric oncology in Germany: results of a population-based retrospective parental survey' *Pediatric Blood & Cancer* 2010, 55(6): 1111–17
6. Antonovsky, A. *Health, Stress and Coping*, Jossey-Bass, San Francisco 1979; and *Unraveling the Mystery of Health*, Jossey-Bass, San Francisco 1987
7. Steiner, R. *Anthroposophy in Everyday Life*, Anthroposophical Press, USA 1995
8. Øgaard, B., Rölla, G. et al. 'Microradiographic study of demineralisation of shark enamel in a human caries model' *Scandinavian Journal of Dental Research* 1988, 96 (3): 209–211
9. Choi, A.L. Sun, G. et al. 'Developmental fluoride neurotoxicity: a systematic review and meta-analysis' *Environmental Health Perspectives* 2012, 120 (10): 1362–1368
10. Pawley, N., Bishop, N.J. 'Prenatal and infant predictors of bone health: the influence of vitamin D' *The American Journal of Clinical Nutrition* 2004, 80 (6): 1748S–1751S; and Zamora, S.A., Rizzoli, R., Belli, D.C. 'Long-term effect of early vitamin-D supplementation on bone mineral status in prematurely born infants' *Journal of Pediatric Gastroenterology and Nutrition* 2000, 31 (1): 94
11. See: www.ncbi.nlm.nih.gov/pmc/articles/PMC3922557; and www.ncbi.nlm.nih.gov/pmc/articles/PMC3896208
12. See www.cdc.gov/mmwr/preview/mmwrhtml/mm6207a4.htm
13. Steiner, R. *Course for Young Doctors*

* **Please note:** some references to specialist medical journals have been omitted from the English version; they can be found in the original German book.

Further Resources

Anthroposophic medicine

Patients and Friends of Anthroposophic Medicine (PAFAM) (UK)
www.pafam.org.uk

Physicians' Association for Anthroposophic Medicine (PAAM) (USA)
paam@anthroposophy.org
www.paam.net

International Federation of Anthroposophic Medical Association (IVAA)
contact@ivaa.info www.ivaa.eu

Sources for medicines

Please note that in some countries some of the medicines mentioned may only be available on prescription, or may have a different name. Try searching online. The following pharmacies may also be able to help:

Buxton & Grant, Bristol, UK
www.buxtonandgrantpharmacy.co.uk

Helios Homeopathy Ltd, Tunbridge Wells, UK
www.helios.co.uk

Uriel Pharmacy Inc. East Troy, USA
www.urielpharmacy.com

Weleda North America
www.weleda.com

Weleda UK Ltd
www.weleda.co.uk

Weleda Australia Pty Ltd
www.weleda.com.au

Weleda New Zealand Ltd
www.weleda.co.nz

Wala stockist UK
www.pharmasana.co.uk

Childbirth, breastfeeding

La Lèche League International
www.LLLi.org

National Childbirth Trust (NCT)
www.nct.org.uk

Waldorf (Steiner) education

Association of Waldorf Schools of North America (AWSNA)
www.waldorfeducation.org

Steiner Waldorf Schools Fellowship (UK)
www.steinerwaldorf.org.uk

Information for other countries can be found through either of the above.

Publications

Steinerbooks
www.steinerbooks.org

Rudolf Steiner Press
www.rudolfsteinerpress.com

Floris Books
www.florisbooks.co.uk

Anthroposophy

Anthroposophical Society in Great Britain
www.anthroposophy.org.uk

Anthroposophical Society in America
www.anthroposophy.org

Anthroposophical Society in Australia
www.anthroposophy.org.au

Anthroposophical Society in Canada
www.anthroposophy.ca

Anthroposophical Society in New Zealand
www.anthroposophy.org.nz

Anthroposophical Society in South Africa
anthroposophysa.org.za

International General Anthroposophical Society
www.goetheanum.org

European Alliance of Applied Anthroposophical Initiatives (ELIANT)
www.eliant.eu

Further Reading

Evans, M. and Rodger, I. *Healing for Body, Soul and Spirit: An Introduction to Anthroposophic Medicine,* Floris Books 2018

Goldberg, R. *Addictive Behaviour in Children and Young Adults,* Floris Books 2012

Gradenwitz-Koehler, E. and Hobbs-Vijendran, M. *Pregnancy, Birth and Beyond: A Spiritual and Practical Guide,* Floris Book 2014

Husemann, A., *The Harmony of the Human Body, Musical Principles in Human Physiology,* Floris Books 2012

Jantzen, C. *Dyslexia: Learning Disorder or Creative Gift?* Floris Books 2009

König, K. *The First Three Years of the Child,* Floris Books 2004

Kornberger, H. *The Power of Stories: Nurturing Children's Imagination and Consciousness,* Floris Books 2008

La Lèche League, *The Womanly Art of Breastfeeding,* La Lèche League International 2010

Lockie, B. *Bedtime Storytelling,* Floris Books 2010

Mellon, N. *Storytelling with Children,* Hawthorn Press 2013

Poplawski, T. *Eurythmy: A Short Introduction to the Art of Movement,* Floris Books 2015

Tapfer, B. and Weisskircher, A. *An Illustrated Guide to Everyday Eurythmy,* Floris Books 2017

Woodward, B. and Hogenboom, M. *Autism, A Holistic Approach,* Floris Books 2013

Index

Gifts and Crafts from Floris Books

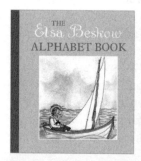

The Elsa Beskow ALPHABET BOOK

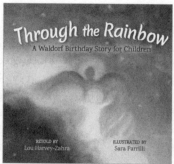

Through the Rainbow
A Waldorf Birthday Story for Children

RETOLD BY
Lou Harvey-Zahra

ILLUSTRATED BY
Sara Parrilli

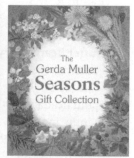

The Gerda Muller Seasons Gift Collection

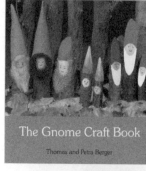

Crafts Through the Year
Thomas and Petra Berger

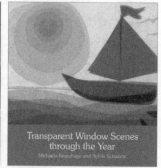

Transparent Window Scenes through the Year
Michaela Kronshage and Sybile Schaarte

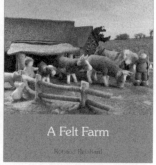

A Felt Farm
Rotraud Reinhard

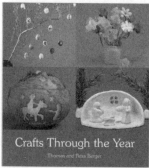

The Gnome Craft Book
Thomas and Petra Berger

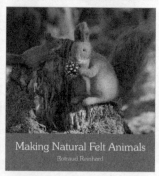

Making Natural Felt Animals
Rotraud Reinhard

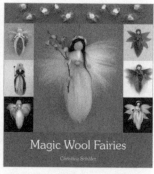

Magic Wool Fairies
Christine Schäfer

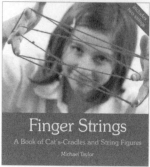

Finger Strings
A Book of Cat's-Cradles and String Figures
Michael Taylor

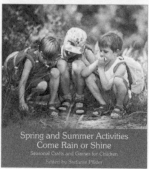

Spring and Summer Activities Come Rain or Shine
Seasonal Crafts and Games for Children
Edited by Stefanie Pfister

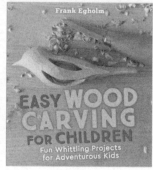

Frank Egholm

EASY WOOD CARVING FOR CHILDREN
Fun Whittling Projects for Adventurous Kids

Parenting Inspiration from Floris Books

Discover our range of practical parenting guides

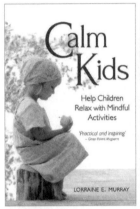

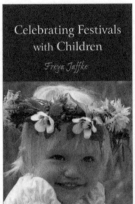

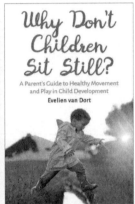

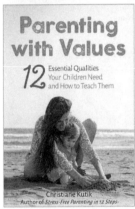

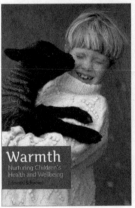

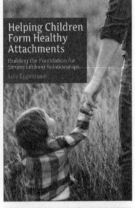

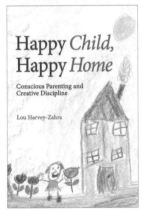

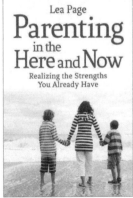

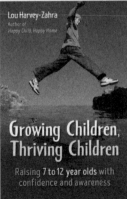

florisbooks.co.uk

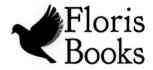

Floris
Books

For news on all our **latest books**,
and to receive **exclusive discounts**,
join our mailing list at:

florisbooks.co.uk

Plus subscribers get a FREE book
with every online order!

We will never pass your details to anyone else.